AF540853

Healing power of HERBS

Dr. S. Suresh Babu
MD (Ayur)
&
Dr. M. Madhavi
B.A.M.S. (MD)

PUSTAK MAHAL®

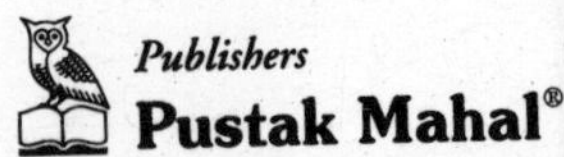

Publishers
Pustak Mahal®

Administrative office and sale centre
J-3/16 , Daryaganj, New Delhi-110002
☎ 23276539, 23272783, 23272784 • *Fax:* 011-23260518
E-mail: info@pustakmahal.com • *Website:* www.pustakmahal.com

Branches
Bengaluru: ☎ 080-22234025 • *Telefax:* 080-22240209
E-mail: pustak@airtelmail.in • pustak@sancharnet.in
Mumbai: ☎ 022-22010941, 022-22053387
E-mail: rapidex@bom5.vsnl.net.in
Patna: ☎ 0612-3294193 • *Telefax:* 0612-2302719
E-mail: rapidexptn@rediffmail.com

© Pustak Mahal, New Delhi

ISBN 978-81-223-0713-9

The book was earlier published under the title
"GREEN REMEDIES – Healing Power of Herbs"

Edition: 2016

NOTICE

The Copyright of this book, as well as all matter contained herein (including illustrations) rests with the Publishers. No person shall copy the name of the book, its title design, matter and illustrations in any form and in any language, totally or partially or in any distorted form. Anybody doing so shall face legal action and will be responsible for damages.

Printed at : Printed at : Rajdhani Book Binding, Delhi

Preface

Acharya Charaka, the great Indian physician and author of 'Charaka-samhita' (the greatest ancient medical classic) says: "The products of a country are most suitable for the treatment of ailments existing in that country". Inspite of this clear cut statement, we under the profound influence of western culture and practices during all these years ignored and neglected our own master's golden and evergreen prescriptions, instructions for perfect health and the effective treatment of ailments with the natural remedies spread-around us.

And once the western thought shifted towards Indian and Chinese medical systems and their rich treasures of natural remedies, we Indians as usual woke-up to rediscover our own belongings under the western lights, proving once again our lack of vision, confidence, and commitment.

As a consequence of this west-east interaction in the field of herbal research, a lot of new information started to pour-in from different quarters. As such an attempt has been made in this work to incorporate all such inputs in addition to the ancient medicinal knowledge. Thus the ancient wisdom and the modern vision are clubbed together to write this small treatise on green remedies in an innovative style to make the work more workable and practical in tune with the saying that science based on nature's laws is eternal. It's value lies in personal experience.

Acknowledgements

These green remedies are gifts of nature, yet many known and unknown people with scientific bend of mind were able to put them in the real practice of healing. We acknowledge all these sources with due respect.

Many of our Post-graduate scholars and colleagues helped us in many ways. We express our sincere thanks to all of them.

We, especially acknowledge the all-round help and support extended by **Dr. P. Jyothi** final year Post graduate scholar in writing and computerizing the book. Without her active involvement this work might not have been completed in time; therefore, our heart-felt thanks to her.

We also acknowledge the help rendered by P G scholar Dr. Dileep Jani, for his share in gathering the vernacular names for a section.

Dr. S. Suresh Babu
MD (Ayu)
&
Dr. M. Madhavi
MD (B.A.M.S.)

Contents

Introduction

Even at its scientific best, modern medicine has its roots in the use of green and herbal remedies. Until 60 years ago nearly all the descriptions of drugs indicated herbal origin in the pharmacopoeia. In the quest for refinement modern chemical technology helped in isolation of the innumerable active principles embedded in those green remedies and such active substances were manufactured synthetically in the laboratories and used as curative agents on the mass-scale in diseased conditions with promising results. After early and initial success these new synthetic magic drugs began to exhibit their inherent drawbacks in the form of adverse side effects during or after their usage. All this has happened because of ignoring the basic natural law the 'in-toto-principle'.

Every herb or green remedy is invariably composed of so many fractions, some are active and dynamic while a few more are passive but are required so that the active component does not harm or damage the human system. This regulatory mode works well if the whole herb or green remedy is consumed in gross form and thereby the safety levels are ensured. Ayurveda , the ancient system of medicine of India which operates on the green herbs/plants/trees etc. also stressed the same. It says that by using, combined herbal preparations rather than using the isolated chemical active ingredients the various chemical constituents will function synergistically and mitigate any harmful side effects.

For instance take the example of the herb ephedrine (simulate); its active ingredient is the alkaloid ephedrine commonly prescribed for treating asthma & cough/bronchitis. The crude plant contains other alkaloids like pseudo-ephedrine that counters the side effects of ephedrine such as increased blood pressure and heartbeat. This can confer relief to an asthma patient if used in total form. Thus a wholesome green plant is nature's gift to the suffering mankind.

Ayurvedic pharmacology known as Dravyaguna utilizes the synergistic cooperation of substances as they co-exist in natural sources. It uses either single plant or more often combinations of plants/herbs as their effects are complimentary. The effectiveness lies in the fact that plants, especially green herbs are concentrated repositories of nature's intelligence which when used properly can increase the expression of that intelligence in the human body.

In this back drop today more and more people are rediscovering the great healing powers of green remedies for their every day health problems. Even in the most advanced countries like USA the demand and sale of green drugs in the name of herbals and health supplements has reached Himalayan heights. The goodness in every layer of the green herbs is creating waves across the globe. A fresh look at the healing powers of green remedies is being undertaken in this book.

Before concluding, we wish to stress the importance of the subject green remedies particularly in Indian context with a thought provoking and trend-setting quotation from "Charaka samhita" the compendium of Indian medicinal knowledge of Ayurveda.

"Yasmin desehi yo jathah tajjam tad aushadham hitham"

[Charaka]

It means that the best medicine for people living in any particular country is the one that grows in that country only. By following this dictum of charaka all the physicians as well as people born in India would do very well if they select or choose their drugs as far as possible from the locality in which they live since the local environment, habit, diet, geographical and climatic factors play a positive role in the treatment. Let us live with plants and grow with green trees.

Dr. S. Suresh Babu
&
Dr. M. Madhavi

Prologue

Herbals—The General Considerations

Holistic or totalistic approach of healing, popularly phrased as holistic medicine, has a bright future in the new millennium despite many dramatic inventions likely to take place in the millennium, for instance, finding longevity genes, harvesting new body parts, inventions of microscopic robots that will enter the blood stream, detect illness, communicate with surgeons and repair cells, high-tech uses of lasers that can now resurface the skin of the aged to restore youthful appearances and repair clogged arteries in the heart or brain etc.

The mind-body-spirit approach of the ancient systems of medicine like India's Ayurveda and China's nature medicine etc. Whatever their lineage, these therapies seem to have certain traits in common. They work gently, slowly in a simpler way, do not harm and can be supplemented along with modern medicine. Moreover these are cost effective and gaining wide-spread acceptance for their effectiveness.

Shifting Trends

The ever increasing demand for the alternative system of healing, over the past 20 years, is due to its grass roots phenomenon. In western countries people pay out of their pockets for these services because insurance still does not cover any thing other than conventional modern medical practices. According to one survey at Stanford University, people who use these alternative medical practices do so because they are :

1. Seeking services of caring practioners who spend time listening to their patients,
2. Seeking treatment for the whole person, not just the sick part of the body.

Further the respondents in the survey, compare much of modern medicine to an impersonal assembly, offering the limited options of drugs with unwanted side effects or surgery. The holistic health concepts do not try to fix the body but instead help super-charge the body's inbuilt healing capacity.

In a nutshell the modern medicine's approach is anti-biotic while the alternative medicine deals in a pro-biotic way.

Major medical institutions of India, Australia, and U.S realizing the importance of the alternative practices are integrating these techniques into their course work and practical experience.

Included in the new line-up of Integrated medicine are :

1. Yoga, relaxation, meditation techniques.
2. Herbal medicine of Ayurveda, China etc.
3. Various therapeutic massage procedures described in ayurveda- upakarma therapy
4. Diet and nutrition.
5. Exercise and movement therapy.
6. Acupuncture.
7. Spirituality.
8. Homoeopathy.

Vision of Health

All the positive shifts taking place in the management of health throughout the globe indicate that health will be a democratic domain and access to affordability, convenience and quality of good care will be realized in the future.

When one faces a catastrophic injury or illness, one will be glad to have the most modern medicine and viable complete services. If one find 'himself with a chronic complaint that most doctors cannot seem to pinpoint then one might just try the resourceful tools of traditional and holistic practioners and be surprised to feel better than ever.

> **One should always remember that vibrant health is not a matter of luck but of smart choices and good living practices. So eat right, exercise, think positive and take time to help others. The future of your health is clean and green.**

The Genesis of Green Herbals

Early man was very close to mother nature, living in daily contact with the plants, animals, mountains, rivers, green valleys; all these were his home. This made him sensitive to these natural things. As such he was able to observe the animals eating many herbal species for their health, for example he noticed that cats eat blades of grass, they digest feathers, hairs and other non digestible matter. These observations led to initiate the early research process in people. Very soon a massive pile up of the medicinal values of the green remedies occurred as a result of these trial and error methods adopted.

This inherited intuitive knowledge of which herb/plant is the right remedy for a particular ailment, is one of the most fascinating aspects of nature and it is not surprising to note that by copying animal, man soon learned how to use nature's healing powers for himself. Thus the knowledge of the green remedies is basically built up on the animal experimentation mode. In a true scientific spirit on becoming more intelligent, man searched for the resemblance of shape of the plant, leaves, seed, roots etc with that of organs of the man, thereby he prescribed heart-shaped leaves for heart problems, kidney shaped nuts for kidney complaints etc. And further from empirical evidence, man acquired knowledge on how plants could do service to him not only for food but also to keep him in good health. In the name of civilization, as people moved away from mother nature, they appeared to have become more prone to disease, decay and degeneration. Because of multiple causes and effects to overcome them, the civilized and urban based man searched for the magic remedies with roots in synthetics and finally procured the much talked antibiotics, steroids etc. These are invaluable gifts to humanity saving lives and improving the quality of existence but only when used with discretion and appropriateness. Without considering the effect on the body systems and the consequences of their indiscriminate use. All this has led to resistance and rebound manifestation of diseases, thereby shifting the focus on to the forgotten natural green remedies once again.

kidney shaped nuts for kidney complaints etc. And further from empirical evidence man acquired knowledge on how plants could be used not only for healing but also to keep him in good health in the name of cultivation. As people moved away from mother nature [illegible] appeared which became more prone to disease, decay and [illegible] because of [illegible] its causes and effects [illegible] the evils of [illegible] and [illegible] man searched for the magic remedies [illegible] in synthetics and finally practised the modern [illegible] no doubt [illegible] gift [illegible] saving lives and improving the quality of [illegible] but only when used with discretion and appropriateness without considering the impact on the body system and the consequences of their indiscriminate use which has brought about a multitude of diseases, thereby shifting the focus on to the [illegible] of the natural green remedies once again.

The Green Approach

The green herbs continue to fascinate man as they have done since the dawn of history. The application of green herbs in many forms to eradicate diseases, remained the corner stone of medical management of different civilizations of the world since time immemorial. Even after the dramatic phenomenal growth of the modern medicine, these herbal practices still continue to flourish.

Some of the major systems of medicine based on green remedies are:-

Ayurveda—the Indian ancient system, Chinese native system, Unani system of Greek origin,Tibet system etc.

Ayurveda and Chinese systems are the most popular among them and the main thrust in this work is on these herbal systems and their green remedies.

On close observation it appears that each system has the things that would be missed by others. What was irrelevant or unwanted information for one practitioner, would be the nucleus for the next. Each somehow captured a different image in its conceptual camera. Each vision had a power and each had blind spots. Therefore an overall review of these proven positive concepts is undertaken in this book to deliver the essence of the systems to the sick person. The competition among medical systems should not be to prove one's superiority over others. The reality of the person and his suffering is of paramount importance.

No system of medicine is perfect, all we can do is an honest exploration of its potentials and limitations and the same is attempted in a humble manner in the following sections of the book. A handshake between all these medical systems can certainly inspire confidence in patients to seek maximum benefits from them.

It is true that we are not giving green remedies a fair chance, we turn to them only as a last resort when all else fails and darkness is there all around.

Well-being and ill-feeling are the two basic factors of the human beings. The dividing line between these two states of health is a very thin as well as sensitive one. Even every minute a small change in the routine of life can cause disharmony of the system, explaining the necessity of the holistic approach in healing care.

The word healing has its roots in the Greek term 'holas' meaning whole and holistic, comprising of physical, psychological, emotional and spiritual components on the same wave length. Herbals too are embedded with numerous vital factors, each factor taking care of a particular component of the (living) human body and it is irrational to extract a chemical from a green plant or herb and throw the rest away. Everything in living nature happens in tune with whole.

The Advantages of the Whole Herb/Plant

A total herb/plant is rarely rapid acting or extremely potents in many chronic diseased conditions. A slow but steady approach is desirable since owing to long drawn pathology of different tissues/organs/systems of the body are in deranged or weakened condition and such continuous bombardment with powerful synthetic drugs is not only undesirable but also dangerous. Therefore a safer and green approach is the right choice as crude preparations of herbs release active ingredients into the blood stream relatively slowly.

The biochemical action of a green herb/drug depends on the totality of the organic and inorganic substances in it. The same active fraction within a plant has remarkably different effects when it is isolated from the plant. It appears that there is some balancing mechanism in the naturally occurring substances of a plant which prevent it from going out of control.

Ayurveda too stresses that disturbance in the balancing state of vata, pitta and Kapha popularly known as tridosha is the main reason for the initiation and production of the disease process. Similarly the Chinese native system too believes that because of disturbances in the balance of 'Yung and Yang' factors, (hot &cold factors) disease occurs . All these are in tune with the basic mechanism of life. This process i.e. balancing act within the body brought back into order by the green remedies like Herbs/plants/ Fruits/Flowers etc because of their inherent balancing action.

There is an in-built regulating effect in herbs and their combinations. For example the most common pungent bulb garlic, can lower the blood pressure of an agitated person known as a Type 'A' Individual and raise the blood pressure if it is low. The active principles derived from this bulb do not possess any such regulatory effect on blood pressure and this is the beauty of the herbals.

Herbals as Tonics

Tonics mean a medication given to stimulate a person who feels run-down or too weak. Herbal tonics generally strengthen the various body tissues, organs and systems by nourishing and toning up the system structurally and functionally without causing any stress to the body. In other words it lubricates and renews the tired system. These herbal tonics are nature's gifts to mankind to maintain health and fitness.

A specific character of these herbal tonics is that they are tender and gentle green remedies that have a mild yet profound effect on the body. Tonic herbs should be separated from curative herbs which are strong in nature; they should be used only in case of diseases in consultation with a herbal doctor. These tonics play a vital role in ensuring that individuals are placed at their peak of health and vitality. The quality of such a positive feeling varies from individual to individual because of many other reasons. Yet everyone can improve the quality of his life with their use.

Gentle Eliminators

There are many green herbals available to be administered orally for purification of the body system. These are usually selected keeping in view the various factors involved in a particular individual. This is the complex problem unique to the herbal practices. Experience, elucidation and experimentation are the tools to acquire the curative power of herbals.

However, the thumb rule is to always use well known and mild herbals. For stimulation and elimination, over active herbals should not be used. There is a possibility of excessive elimination of body fluids along with body's internal toxins which may cause unpleasant situations.

The following are some suggestions for herbals that are effective and safer. This is not the comprehensive list but simply the examples to point the way:-

1. **Adaptogenic**	a substance that regulate the production of hormones	1. Ashwagandha. 2. Shatavari.
2. **Alterative**	helps in the restoration of the general well being.	1. Tinospora/Indian gooseberry.
3. **Anti Microbal Infective**	helps to fight off infective organisms.	1. Neem. 2. Tulasi. 3. Garlic.
4. **Diaphoretic**	helps in sweating, to remove toxins from the skin.	1. Tulasi. 2. Castor plant roots.
5. **Diuretic**	helps in promoting the urine flow.	1. Barley water. 2. Coconut water. 3. Punarnava. 4. Gokshur.
6. **Expectorant**	helps in removal of excess mucus from the lungs.	1. Yasti. 2. Vibhetaki.
7. **Hepatic**	helps in detoxifying the liver.	1. Katuki 2. Bhuamlaki. 3. Bhringraj.
8. **Laxative**	helps in mobilising the bowels.	1. Sena leaves. 2. Green fibrous food. 3. Castor oil (Medicinal). 4. Trivrutt.
9. **Tonic**	helps to promote health.	1. Amla. 2. Harad. 3. Ashwagandha

Basic Ayurvedic Concepts

- According to ayurveda the ancient Indian medical science 'health is an indication of normal biological processes which would help maintain mental and physical alertness and happiness'
- Disease could develop from body and mind due to exogenous and natural intrinsic causes.
- Treatment of diseases means use of drugs, control of diet and involves practices for recovery of health.

It is amazing to find how even in the ancient times, the Indian Material medical could classify drugs based on their physiological actions and specify the details of the habitat of different plants, the parts to be used and the proper time for their collection, method of storage etc. It is thus abundantly clear that the users of the ayurvedic system were fully aware of the important factors regulating the yield of active principles and the efficacy of the drug preparation. It is equally interesting to note that during that period chemistry of natural products isolated both from flora and fauna was also developed.

Thus organic compounds were divided into two broad classes, vegetable and animal. The former includes fermented oral liquids, juices of plants, fruits and plant tissues while honey, milk, curd, butter, etc. were the animal substances. The major interest was however centered around the applications of these vegetable and animal compounds in the manufacture of medicines.

It is no wonder that the reputation of the system of healing science spread far and wide and attracted the attention of the contemporary civilized nations. In the Greek and Roman medicine. For instance, many herbal remedies, e.g. smoking of datura in cases of asthma, use of nux vomica in paralysis, application of opium in diarrhoea etc. found prominent place in the works of these medicinal systems.

- **Dosha** — According to ayurveda the entire biological process of the living organism is governed by three essential factors viz., vata, pitta and sleshma which are singularly called dosha and grouped together as tridoshas. Abnormalities or maladies are considered to be the effects of imbalance in the tridoshas.

- **Tridosha**

  1. Vata: It explains all the biological phenomena which are controlled by the functions of the central and autonomic nervous systems. The malfunction of vata is the major factor in developing diseases either by itself or coupled with other functional disorders due to pitta and kapha.
  2. Pitta: It is the manifestation of energy (Tejas) in the living organisms that helps digestion, assimilation, tissue building, heat production, blood-pigmentation, activeness of the endocrine glands and so on.

3. Kapha (sleshma): It implies the functions of thermostasis or heat regulation and also formation of various preservative fluids e.g.- mucus, synovial etc. The main function of kapha is to provide nutrition to body-tissues, to bring about co-ordination of body-systems and regulation of all biological processes.

Basis of Drug-action

I. Rasa: is based on taste. Different types of tastes of herbal drugs are considered to induce various physiological activities in the body depending on their constituents. The types of tastes are—

1. Madhura (sweet)
2. Amla (sour)
3. Lavana (salty)
4. Katu (Pungent)
5. Tikta (Bitter)
6. Kasaya (Astringent)

1. Madhura Rasa: Pleasant, brain and heart tonic, galactogogue i.e. promotes secretion of milk and other fluids.

2. Amla Rasa: Appetizer and digestive, sialagogue.

3. Lavana Rasa: Readily soluble, water-retaining, softening, appetizer, digestive expectorant, diuretic.

4. Katu Rasa: Sialagogue, appetizer, lacrimatory and produces tingling sensation on tongue, useful in dyspepsia.

5. Tikta Rasa: Appetizer, produces dryness in the mouth.

6. Kasaya Rasa: Healing of wounds, diuretic, causes stiffness and soreness of throat and dryness in mouth.

Relationship Between Rasa & Tridosha

Rasa	Vata	Pitta	Kapha
Madhura	Pacifies	Pacifies	Aggravates
Amla	Pacifies	Aggravates	Aggravates
Lavana	Pacifies	Aggravates	Aggravates
Katu	Aggravates	Aggravates	Pacifies
Tikta	Aggravates	Pacifies	Pacifies
Kasaya	Aggravates	Pacifies	Pacifies

Vipaka

Metabolism of the products arising out of the biochemical changes of food and drugs during the gastro-intestinal digestion, is called Vipaka.

Difference in Action between Rasa and Vipaka

Rasa	**Vipaka**
Immediate	Delayed
Local	Systemic
Physiological & Psychological	Physiological
Perceivable	Non-perceivable, Inferable.

Veerya

The potency of a drug (clinical efficacy) is of two types:

Sheeta	**Ushna**
Diminishes secretions	Storing up of energy
Stabilises excretory functions	Easy digestion
Stops bleeding	Thirst-causing
Promotes Vigour, vitality	Aggravates pitta
Aggravates vata and kapha doshas	Pacifies vata, kapha
Pacifies pitta	

Prabhava

Prabhava refers to specific characteristic influence of a drug that cannot be explained otherwise (empirical action).

Guna

Denotes the physical properties of the drug. These are twenty in number.

1. **Guru (Heavy):** Induces the feeling of heaviness, dullness, fatigue, promotes quantity of waste products, impairs the digestion.
2. **Lagu (Light):** Promotes fitness of the body, helps in easy digestion.
3. **Sheeta (Cold):** Cooling effect, promotes vata and kapha doshas, pacifies pitta impedes blood flow.
4. **Ushna (Hot):** Increases body temperature, causes thirst, aggravates pitta, improves blood circulation, increases urine and sweat, stimulates appetite and digestion.
5. **Snigdha (Unctuous):** Produces soothing effect on the body, pacifies vata, promotes kapha and eliminates waste products.
6. **Ruksha (Dry):** Uncomfortable feeling, reduces vigor, vitality and libido.

7. **Manda (Dull):** Acts slowly and pacifies deranged dosha.
8. **Teekshna (Sharp):** Rapid acting, potent, clears the body channels, removes morbidity and aggravates pitta.
9. **Sthira (Immobile):** Stabilizes the physiological functions .
10. **Sara (Spreading):** Penetrative, stimulates excretory system.
11. **Mrudu (Soft):** Makes body tissues soft and loose. Increases kapha and pacifies vata, pitta.
12. **Kathina (Hard):** Causes stiffness and firmness of the body and excites vata.
13. **Vishada (Clear):** Removes sliminess, promotes vata and heals ulcers.
14. **Picchila (Slim):** Increases body weight, promotes fracture & wound healing and stimulates excretory organs.
15. **Slakshna (Smooth):** Promotes tissue synthesis, increases kapha and pitta.
16. **Khara (Rough):** Leads to emaciation, aggravates vata.
17. **Sthula (Bulky):** Not easily digestible, obstructs vessels, tubes and channels of the body.
18. **Sukshma (Minute):** Penetrates all parts of the body and stimulates vata.
19. **Sandra (Solid):** Which nourishes the body.
20. **Drava (Fluid):** Pervades the entire body.

According to ayurveda all the herbals and other remedies exhibit their actions on the basis of the essential factors as explained above.

Charaka Samhita — The authentic text of ayurveda, classified plants/herbals into 50 groups based on their chief physiological actions in the body. It is one of the rare scientific explorations taken place in ancient India.

Advantages of Ayurveda

- It is preventive, protective, health promotive and curative in nature. At the same time herbal remedies are self-contained, and nutritive rendering them harmless and non-toxic.

  This provides a constructive approach against destructive forces.
- Ayurveda is not man-made but is believed to be a divine gift. It is for us to study, seek search and take the benefits from this treasure of knowledge.
- Ayurveda is mainly based on herbs, plants, flowers, fruits, vegetables and all vegetation that grows around us in plenty. It is our native system based on the peculiar Indian conditions. Further whatever is available in our own country

is bound to be more suitable in creating good health to us rather than borrowed knowledge as well as materials. Charaka samhita stresses the same point.

- Ayurveda begins when everything fails and when the treatment is uncertain and prolonged, ayurvedic approach is the right choice since it cures chronic and stubborn diseases by its deep-rooted treatment procedures and drugs.

Tibetan Medical System

The fundamental concepts of Tibetan medical system, like ayurveda, revolves around the five cosmo physical energies and three humoral energies. The working concepts of Ayurveda like pancha bhutas, tri-doshas, sapta-dhatus, mala traya etc. also constitute the main features of Tibetan medicine.

Pulse diagnosis and urine analysis also form the distinctive feature of Tibetan system. The most unique feature of Tibetan medicine is its integrated buddhist approach to mind and body. Ignorance and three in-born mental poisons such as attachment, anger and delusions are the main cause of all sufferings, it believes.

The history of Tibetan medical system dates back some 3,800 years to the time of the non-buddhist culture of Tibet's native religion "DON". It has continued to evolve since then to the time of the strong emergence of buddhist culture in India.

The Tibetans made use of their country's abundant natural resources of flora and fauna to fight against diseases. The 7th and 8th century A.D saw real development in the field of Tibetan medicine. Ayurveda has contributed a great deal in enriching the system.

The Gyud-shi or the four great classics which are most authoritative texts of Tibetan medicine bear ample proof of its loyal alleigance to ayurvedic classics like Charaka, Sushruta Samhitas and Astanga Hrudaya.

The Unani System

The Unani System, is based on the humoral theory which supposes the presence of four humors in our body.

1. Blood
2. Phlegm
3. Yellow Bile and
4. Black Bile

People's temperaments like sanguine, phlegmatic, choleric and melancholic coincide with the preponderance of these humors respectively.

Blood is hot and moist, phlegm is cold and moist, yellow bile is hot and dry and black bile is cold and dry. The basic principles of Unani system are similar with that of ayurveda. Unani system believes that every person has a unique humoral constitution which represents his healthy state. Any change in it affects his health.

There is a power of self-preservation or adjustment called the defence mechanism which strives to restore disturbances within the limits prescribed by the constitution of an individual.

The Unani system is the result of the fusion of diverse thoughts and experiences of nations with an ancient cultural heritage, like Egypt, Iraq, Iran, India, Arabia and China. Unani originated in the 5th and 4th centuries BC under the patronage of Hippocrates in Greece.

Chinese System of Medicine

The Chinese native system of medicine is also like Ayurveda, and dates back to ancient times. The entire Chinese system revolves around the classical work "Nei-ching" by Huang Ti (2598BC).

Basic Points

1. According to it, the human body is made up of five elements—Wood, Fire, Earth, Metal and Water.
2. The Materia Medica is very rich with many vegetable, animal and mineral remedies. The great pharmacopoeia "pen-though kangamu" spread over 52 volumes, was compiled first time in 1552. Since then it has been revised many a times and is still considered an authority on Chinese drugs.
3. Acupuncture, the Needle Therapy, is one of the most popular therapies of China, even accepted by the western cultures. It is now widely practised throughout the world without any reservation, just like the "yoga" of ancient India.

Herbal Medicine Pharmacology

Herbal medical pharmacology cannot be explained in terms of modern pharmacological Scrutinising methods. It has got its own basis; for instance, in Ayurveda, each drug has got distinct features like Rasa, Guna, Veerya, Vipaka and Prabhava differing from one part of the plant to the other.

The therapeutic potency of individual drugs varies according to the place, season and time of collection of the raw drug and the form in which the medicines are dispensed i.e. Kashaya (decoction), Gutika (pill), Arista (alcoholic oral liquid) etc.

According to their therapeutic efficacy and features, the drugs are grouped in different categories or Vargas. A particular Varga (group) is selected for the treatment of diseases of a particular system (see box above).

There should be compatibility between the drug qualities and doshas predominant in a patient to obtain maximum therapeutic efficiency. As such Ayurvedic pharmacology therapy is more individualized and not generalised as in the case of modern medicine.

"Pathya"—The Food-drug Interactions

The food-drug and drug-drug interactions are well known to our ancient physicians, which is why certain foodstuff, drinks, regimen etc were prohibited during the treatment. This food-drug theory is known as "Pathya-Apathya" in Ayurveda, which means that when a patient is put on a particular drug regimen, he has to totally avoid certain foodstuff, for instance, Ayurveda restricts intake of tamarind with mineral preparations, since tamarind contains tannins and tartaric acid, which will reduce the absorption of minerals.

Further, the restrictions imposed on the patients in the name of "pathya" in fact are evolved to protect the human system from potent drugs which may cause injury or irritation.

2.

The Green Pharmacy

Collecting Herbs

Introduction

The collection of required green herbs is a pleasant exercise, if one does have a positive attitude towards the natural things in life. Searching out herbs in the open nature offers an opportunity to know the richness of the botanical wealth available around us. We live in a natural world that promotes the process of healing, a world that contains herbs beneficial to man.

Even though there are many details about the collection and process of herbs described in Ayurvedic and other herbal systems of medicine, the heart of the matter is the consciousness that is brought to it by the collector of the drug.

Research studies made many contributions regarding the plant chemistry, active principles, growing the herbs etc. All these developments once again prove the solid basis of Ayurvedic principles regarding picking up of the particular type of plant at a prescribed time/season.

Some general observations on procurement of herbs/plants :

1. The curative or active principles embedded in herbs are at peak level, before the end of active growth. As such plants should be picked up just on their opening into blossom.
2. A day without rain is ideal for collecting.
3. In the case of leaves only best shaped and green leaves should be gathered, and the leaves that are withered, insect-bitten or stained should be discarded.

Ayurveda recommends the collection of herbs in the following way:

When to Collect 'Green Herbs'

Parts of Herb	Season of Collection
1. Moola i.e. Root	Greshma, Shishira. (Summer, Early Winter)
2. Patra/Leaves	Varsha, Vasantha. (Monsoon, Spring)
3. Kanda/Branches	Varsha/Vasanta. (Monsoon, Spring)
4. Pushpa/Flowers	Flowering season
5. Phala/Fruits	Seasonal

6. Sara/Plant marrow	Hemantha (Winter)
7. Twak/Bark	Sharat (Autumn)
8. Kanda/Tuber	Sharat (Autumn)
9. Ksheera/Milk	Sharat (Autumn)
10. Pancha Angas/Whole Plant	Sharat (Autumn)

4. The leaves and herbs should be cut with a sharp steel knife. Pulling the leaves by hand may easily damage the tender stems of the plant, which in turn may cause delay in regrowth of the plant or it may lead to the entry of fungus or insects into the damaged tissue of plant.
5. Many important green herbs, plants, grow on the waste-lands, grave yard, road side etc. but while gathering, these phaces should be avoided, and plants from cleaner surrounding areas only should be picked-up for medicinal purpose.

Herbs Unfit for Use

The following types of herbs/plants should not be collected.

- Plants from fields sprayed with agro chemicals as they will dry along with the herbs.
- Herbs grown in polluted areas like chemically treated tanks, canals etc. should be avoided.

Most of the herbs are grown seasonally and they should be collected in the right season and preserved carefully for future use. Drying herbs is one of the easiest ways in this regard; moreover drying also acts as a preservative. It keeps up the quality of the drug.

The Method of Drying Herbs

Green herbs collected should be dried in shade by spreading them in loose, single layers on flat drying surfaces like wooden tables etc. Wire cooling racks used in kitchen are of special use, since they allow air circulation underneath and quicker drying. Therefore drying depends on the herbs and the environment and requires a regular check-up.

Three Easy Steps of Roots Drying

- To dry up roots, first unearth them gently, wash the root to remove all dirt and dust and scrub well with a nailbrush if necessary.
- Cut off tops and trim away rootlets. If it is a large root, slice it up into strips about 5cm long, depending on the root.
- Spread the stripes out on a drying rack and leave in a warm place for 10 to 15 days turning them over daily.

Note: To dry bulbs and corns, tie them up in small bunches like onions in a shed. Keep constant watch to see that they are drying evenly.

Storing Herbs

When the herbs are dried-up properly the immediate task is to store them properly so as to preserve the medicinal properties ascribed to them. Dried herbs, whether root or aerial part should be placed immediately in a dry container.

Any herb which contains volatile oils should not be stored in ordinary plastic boxes or sacks, instead they should be placed in glazed ceramic, dark-glass or metal containers with tight-fitting lids.

When to Acquire Green Herbs

In every season nature gifts away some medicinally useful herbs, plants, flowers, fruits etc. Following is the guide for collection of herbs and their individual parts. The information tabulated is general in nature; local conditions will vary from region to region.

Harvesting Seasons of Certain Important Green Remedies.

Drug	Parts/used	Season
Ajwoin	Dried Ripe Fruit	May/June
Aniseed	Dried Ripe Fruit	Jan/Apr
Cardamom	Ripe Fruit	Aug/Jan
Chillies	Ripe Fruit	Apr/Jun, Sep/Dec
Clove	Unopened Flower	Nov/Feb
Coriander	Dried/Mature Fruits	July/Aug, Nov/Mar
Cumin Seeds	Dried Seeds	Feb/Apr
Dil Seeds	Seeds	jan/Feb
Fennel	Dried Ripe Fruits	Feb/Apr
Fenugreek	Dried Ripe Fruits	Feb/Apr
Garlic	Bulb	Dec/Mar
Ginger	Rhizome	Nov/Dec
Mustard	Dried Seeds	Dec/May
Onion	Bulb	Mar/May
Black Pepper	Dried Berries	Nov/Mar
Saffron	Dried Stigma	Oct/Nov
Tamarind	Dried Fruits	Apr/May
Himalayan Silver Fir	Dried Leaves	Mar/Jun
Turmeric	Dried Rhizomes	Dec/Feb
Khaskhas	Dried Seeds	Nov

Green Pharmacy/Forms of Remedies

Green remedies are generally used in two forms:

1. As internal remedies in diseases like fever, cough, diarrhoea etc. in the form of powder, tablets, decoction, infusions etc.
2. As external remedies for application in complaints like injuries, swellings and other skin diseases in the form of medicinal oils, ointments, poultice etc.

Therefore the method of preparation of all these types of herbal remedies is described in this chapter in an easy-to-make manner.

Internal Remedies

The most effective way of using herbs is to administer them internally, as many health problems including those appearing externally have roots inside the body. The methods of preparation of herbal remedies are numerous, yet these can be classified under 3 broad categories.

- Water based extracts.
- Alcohol based extracts.
- Fresh and dry herbs.

Water Based Preparation

These preparations can be made by everybody at home in two ways: infusions and decoctions. When the herbs to be used consist of any hard or woody material "decoction" method is the right medium, while for the herbs which are fresh and green "infusion" is used.

Infusion: Infusions are most suitable for plant parts such as fresh leaves, flowers, seeds or resin by making a coarse powder, so that the cell walls of these are broken and made accessible to the water medium.

Seeds, such as fennel and aniseed should be slightly bruised before being used in an infusion to release the volatile oils from the cells. Any aromatic herb should be infused in a pot that has a well-sealed lid to ensure that only a minimum of the volatile oil is lost during the process of exportation.

Cold Infusion: When the herbs/other parts of the plant to be used are sensitive to heat, due to rich content of volatile substances or because their constituents break down at high temperature, cold infusions of these materials is the appropriate measure.

The ratio of drug/herb to that of water is the same but in this case the infusion should be left over for 6 to 1 2 hours in a well-sealed earthen pot. When the liquid is ready, strain and use it.

The Making of Infusions

1. Take a clean glass or steel teapot, put one or two teaspoons full of the dried herb or herbal mixture (as recommended) into it, keeping in view the quantity of the infusion you want to make.
2. Pour a cup or cups (as recommended) of boiling water into the pot and leave the lid on for 10 to 15 minutes. Then filter the infusion into a cup in recommended quantity and drink once or twice a day as prescribed.
   - Infusion may be drunk hot, which is normally best for medicinal herbs.
   - In case the infusion is too bitter to drink, it can be sweetened with liquorice root powder or honey or sugar syrup. (Diabetics should not use them)

The Preparation of Green Remedies

Most of the plants, herbs and herbals are administered in the following forms:

- **Fresh Juice/Swarasa:** The expressed juice of fresh leaves, flowers, bark, root etc. The fresh tender parts are ground well then pressed for extraction of juice. This, if one desires, can be filtered through a clean cloth. Since these are bitter in taste to make it palatable one can add honey or syrup to it. However for diabetic patients, honey or sugar should not be added. In case the drug is in dry form, it should be well soaked in water for some time before it can be ground.

- **Paste/Kalka:** It is the form of medicine, wherein the herb or needed parts of the plant is made into a paste by constantly adding some water or milk. For fresh green herbs no water should be added as they contain sufficient quantity of water.

- **Decoction**: Wash the drug to remove the unwanted dirt, dust etc. Then chop it into small pieces and pound well. Boil 1/2 cup of the drug in 4 cups of water (1:8) and reduce it to one cup. Filter the decoction and use.

- **Herbal Tea**: Make the coarse powder of the required drug material and mix 1 to 2 teaspoons full of the powder to 1 and 1/2 cups of water and boil till it is reduced to one cup. Add sugar or honey and drink.

- **Powder**: Dry up the required drug materials well in the shade, away from direct sunlight. Grind or crush it and sieve through a fine cloth to obtain a fine powder of the desired drug.

- **Syrup**: Pure honey or sugar can be used to preserve liquid medicines like decoctions and infusions. Syrups are ideally suited for children and delicate persons, who cannot tolerate bitter medicines. Cough syrups, liver syrups, fever syrups and antidiarrhoeal syrups are more common. Honey is particularly soothing.

Method of Preparation

Heat 200 ml infusion or decoction in a clean steel vessel. Add 200 grams of pure honey or sugar and stir continuously until dissolved completely.

Allow the mixture to cool and pour into a dark glass bottle. Seal with a cork stopper. The cork is important as syrups often ferment and screw-capped bottles can explode.

Items Required for Syrup Preparation

200ml liquid medicine (decoction or infusion), 200 grams honey or sugar, steel spoon, dark glass bottle with cork stoppers.

General Dosage: 5 to 15 ml thrice a day.

Cream

A cream is a mixture of water with fats or oils which soften and blend with the skin. It can be easily made using emulsifying ointment, which is a mixture of oils and waxes that blend with water.

Home made cream will last for couple of months but the shelf life is prolonged by storing the mixture in a cool place or refrigerator or by adding a few drops of benzoin tincture or by adding 100mg vitamin C, a safe and good preservative.

Methods of Preparation

- Melt the fats or wax and water in a bowl over a pan of boiling water, add the herbal paste and heat gently for 2 hours.
- Stir well and strain the mixture into a bowl. Stir constantly until it becomes cold.
- Use a small steel knife to fill into jars or bottle; put some cream around the edge of the jar first and then fill the middle.

Ointment

Ointments contain only oils or fats but no water, and unlike creams they do not blend with the skin but form a separate layer over it. Ointments are suitable where the skin is already weak or soft or where some protection is required. Once, ointments were prepared with animal fat but petroleum jelly (Vaseline) or paraffin wax is the suitable medium now.

Methods of Preparation

- Melt the wax or jelly in a bowl over a pan of boiling water, stir in the herbal paste and heat for about one hour or until it becomes crisp.
- Pour the mixture into a jelly bag or a cloth fitted with an elastic band which is held over the rim of a jug.
- Wear rubber gloves as the mixture is very hot and squeeze it through the jelly bag into the jug.

- Quickly pour the strained mixture while it is still warm and molten, into clean glass storage jars.

Powder and Capsules

Herbs can be consumed as powders well mixed into water or sprinkled on food or filled into capsules. Capsules are preferred generally when the drug powder is very bitter in taste and unpalatable. Another advantage of capsule form is that it can be carried around. However, it is best to use commercially prepared powders which are available in the herbal medical stores. Grinding herbs in a domestic grinder generates heat, which can cause chemical changes in the herbs and hard roots and can damage the grinder. Two part gelatin empty capsules are available in medical stores.

Home Capsule Filling Method

To fill capsules, pour the herbal powder into a clean steel saucer, separate the two halves of a capsule case and slide them together through the powder scooping it into the capsule.

Fit together the two halves of the capsule and store in a dark glass jar in a cool place.

Compress: A compress is simply a cloth pad soaked in a hot herbal extract and applied to the painful area for sometime. A cold compress is used for headaches.

Method

- Soak a clean piece of soft cloth in a hot infusion or other herbal extracts and squeeze out the excess liquid.
- Hold the pad against the area. When it cools or dries, repeat the process using a hot mixture.

Poultice: Poultice has a similar action to a compress, but here the whole herb rather than a liquid extract is applied. Poultices are generally applied hot.

Method

- Boil the fresh herb, squeeze out any surplus liquid and spread it on to the area. Apply a little oil on the skin first to prevent the herb from sticking.
- Apply gauze or cotton strips to hold the poultice carefully in place.

Parts of Plants Used in Remedies

1. Androecium, 2. Anther, 3. Aril, 4. Bulb, 5. Dry Fruit, 6. Dry seed, 7. Exudate, 8. Endosperm, 9. Flower, 10. Fruit, 11. Fruit Rind, 12. Fruit Pulp, 13. Gall, 14. Heart Wood, 15. Inflorescence, 16. Leaf, 17. Latex, 18. Oil, 19. Plant (Whole), 20. Root, 21. Root Bark, 22. Root Tuber, 23. Rhizome, 24. Seed, 25. Seed coat, 26. Stem, 27. Stem Bark, 28. Stem Tuber, 29. Style & Stigma, 30. Resin.

• [illegible] pour the strained mixture [illegible] into [illegible] storage jars.

Powder and Capsules

Herbs can be [illegible] as powders [illegible] water [illegible] into capsules. Capsules are [illegible] the [illegible] however [illegible] medical stores.

Home Capsule Filling Method

To fill capsules, place the herbal powder into a clean [illegible] halves of a capsule [illegible] the capsule.

• Fit together the two halves of the capsule [illegible]

Compress: A compress is [illegible]

Method

• Soak a clean piece of [illegible] extracts and [illegible]

• Hold the pad against the area [illegible]

Poultice: [illegible] has a similar action to a compress but [illegible]

Method

• Boil the fresh herb [illegible] and spread it on to the [illegible]

• [illegible]

Parts of Plants Used in Remedies

1. [illegible] 2. [illegible] 3. [illegible] 4. [illegible] 5. [illegible] 6. [illegible] 7. [illegible] 8. [illegible] 9. [illegible] 10. [illegible] 11. [illegible] 12. [illegible] 13. [illegible] 14. [illegible] 15. [illegible] 16. [illegible] 17. [illegible] 18. [illegible] 19. [illegible] 20. [illegible] 21. [illegible] 22. [illegible] 23. [illegible] 24. [illegible] 25. [illegible] 26. [illegible] 27. [illegible] 28. [illegible] 29. [illegible] 30. [illegible]

3.

GREEN REMEDIES—INDIVIDUAL PROFILES

1. Ajowan (Ajmud)

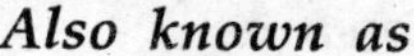

Also known as

Latin	Carum roxburghianum
English	Ajowan
Sanskrit	Ajamoda
Hindi	Ajmud
Marathi	Ajmoda
Tamil	Asamtavoman
Telugu	Ajumoda, vamu
Malayalam	Ayamodhakam
Kannada	Ajamodhavoma

How it looks—It is an erect branched annual herb with bipinnate leaves, white flowers and oval fruits.

What we use—fruits

What it does—It is thermogenic, antispasmodic, stimulant, digestive, carminative and anthelmintic.

How we use it—

In **flatulence**—Take a tsp of ajowan seeds and roast it in a pan until the seeds turn red. Pour 2 cups of water into the pan and boil until the water is reduced to half. Take this decoction once a day for a safe and sure remedy for gaseous distension of the abdomen.

In **common cold**—To clear a nasal block, crush a tsp of ajowan and tie in a cloth bundle for inhaling. The strong odour soon clears the stuffy nose.

In **asthma**—Inhale the vapours of a tsp of the seeds put in boiling water.

In **earache**—Half a tsp of ajowan is heated in half a glass of milk and the milk is filtered and used as ear drops.

In **sprains**—Mix a paste of ajowan, salt and turmeric in gingelly oil and apply on the sprained area along with some wheat flour.

In **worms**—Make a powder of seeds. Mix 2-tsp of powder with black salt in equal amount and take in night with water.

In **gout**—Make a powder of seeds and take 2/3-tsp with warm milk three times a day.

In **kidney pain**—Make powder of seeds. Take 2-tsp in the morning and evening with warm milk.

2. Almond (Badam)

Also known as

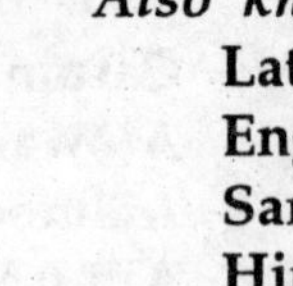

Latin	:	**Prunus dulcis**
English	:	**Almond**
Sanskrit	:	**Vatadah**
Hindi	:	**Badam**
Marathi	:	**Badam**
Tamil	:	**Vatamkottai**
Telugu	:	**Badam vittulu**
Malayalam	:	**Badamkotta**
Kannada	:	**Badami**

How it looks—It is a middle sized tree with simple greyish leaves (when Mature) and white-tinged red, showy flowers. The fruits are velvetty drupes, separating into 2 halves, exposing stones which contain the kernel called almond.

What we use—Kernel, oil

What it does—*Kernel*—Sweet thermogenic, aphrodisiac, laxative, diuretic, nutritious, demulcent and nervine tonic.

Oil—Sweet, cooling, antispasmodic, sedative, laxative, rejuvenating.

How we use it—

In **delayed puberty**—Crush a few almonds, along with egg yolk, gingelly powder and a tsp of honey in milk and give it to the girl with delayed onset of puberty, every day. This ensures good overall development during adolescence.

In **pregnancy**—Almonds being highly nutritive are an ideal source of energy for pregnant women. For best results, soak almonds in milk, add a pinch of saffron and drink the tasty preparation everyday for nourishment both to the mother and the to-be child.

To **increase vitality**—Almonds in milk also increase libido and enhance general sexual performance in cases of frigidity too.

As a **brain tonic**—Almond is popular for its property as a nervine tonic. Rich in nourishment and essential fats, almonds serve to enhance memory and intelligence. Soak 4-6 almonds in water and eat after removing the kernel.

As **a body coolant**—Badam kheer is a well known preparation made by grinding almonds and mixing in milk. This cools the body apart from relieving brain exhaustion and improving functioning.

As it contains copper and iron, it helps in synthesising blood haemoglobin.

As it is a potent aphrodisiac, its regular use increases sexual power.

3. Aloe (Ghritkumari)

Also known as

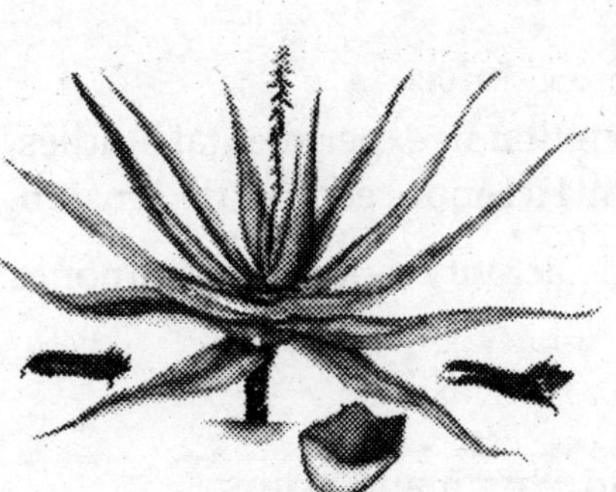

Latin	**:**	**Aloe Vera**
English	**:**	**Aloe**
Sanskrit	**:**	**Kumari**
Hindi	**:**	**Ghritkumari**
Marathi	**:**	**Korafad**
Tamil	**:**	**Kattalai**
Telugu	**:**	**Kalabanda**
Malayalam	**:**	**Kattuvala**
Kannada	**:**	**Kathaligidi**

How it looks—It is a coarse perennial with a short stem and shallow root system. The leaves are fleshy with horny prickles on the margins, and the flowers are yellow or orange in colour.

What we use—Leaf juice

What it does—It is bitter, cooling, anthelmintic, carminative, diuretic, stomachic and emmenagogue.

How we use it—

In **jaundice**—A few drops of aloe juice is instilled in the nostrils to control jaundice.

In **liver disorders and splenomegaly**—Aloe juice with turmeric powder should be taken twice a day to combat these conditions.

In **difficult urination**—In high fever, sometimes, this condition arises. Consume diluted aloe juice from time to time to alleivate this condition.

In **wounds**—Boil aloe leaves and take the fleshy part of the inside of the leaves to use as a poultice over wounds.

In **burning sensation**—Paste cumin seeds with aloe juice and apply over the area. Even in burns, the above mixture may be applied from time to time to hasten healing and prevent scar formation.

As a **cosmetic**—Aloe is one of the best known moisturisers and is used freely in creams and shampoos to retain moisture in skin and hair.You can make your own home-made moisturiser and cleanser in the following way—

Take ½ tsp of lemon juice and ½ tsp of aloe juice. Dilute this with about 4 tsp of water. After filtering apply this mixture over the face and neck and wash off after 15 minutes.

Modern Studies

1. Aloe was found to significantly inhibit gastric acid secretion in experimental studies, and was thereby seen to protect gastric mucosa from Hcl-induced gastric tension.
2. The aqueous extract of aloe also exhibited antiparasitic activity against trichomonas vaginalis, a vaginal fungus.
3. Aloe is found to be good against Piles.
4. Aloe is also found to be soothing for arthritis and rheumatic pains.
5. It is also found to be of high value in treating blood dysentery.

4. Arjun (Arjun)

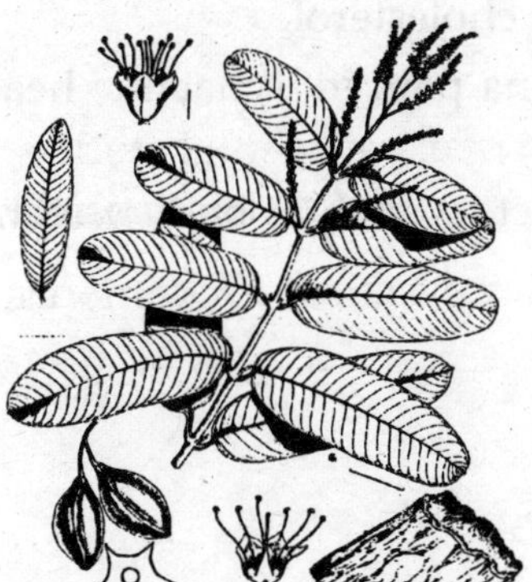

Also known as

Latin	:	**Terminalia arjuna**
English	:	**Arjun**
Sanskrit	:	**Arjunah**
Hindi	:	**Arjun**
Marathi	:	**Srdhaval**
Tamil	:	**Attumarutu**
Telugu	:	**Erramaddi**
Malayalam	:	**Nirmaruta**
Kannada	:	**Maddi**

How it looks—It is a large evergreen tree with a spreading crown and drooping branches. The bark is smooth grey and buttressed. The flowers are white and the fruits ovoid with 5-1 hard angles curving upwards.

What we use—Bark

What it does—Astringent, cooling, aphrodisiac, demulcent, cardiotonic, styptic, antidysenteric, urinary astringent, expectorant and tonic.

How we use it—

As a **cardiac tonic**—It is a highly esteemed cardiac toxic and a preparation called "Arjuna Ksheera Paka" is repeatedly used with encouraging results in the Ayurvedic medical field. Here is how you prepare it.

Add 2 tsp of Arjun bark powder to a glass of milk diluted with 4 glasses of water. Boil this preparation down to a glass. Take this in two doses everyday to keep your heart fit and ward off problems of angina, cholesterol and high blood pressure.

In **wounds**—Make a decoction of the bark powder and wash wounds with it. This aids the healing process and speedens normalisation of skin.

In **fractures**—Take a tsp of the powder of the bark everyday to facilitate quick healing of bone tissue in fractures.

In **diabetes**—Taking a decoction of the bark everyday is very useful in diabetes as the tannins contained in the bark tone the endocrine system.

As a **cosmetic**—In spotty and discoloured skin, make a face pack of the bark powder and milk and use everyday to lighten spots and patches.

Modern Studies

1. It has been observed that Arjuna bark powder in doses of 20mg/100mg of body weight brings about a significant reduction in plasma cholesterol.
2. Another study has confirmed that Arjuna alleviates angina pain in ischaemic heart disease patients and patients with rhythm disturbances.
3. The drug also appears to modify known coronary risk factors such as body weight, blood pressure, blood sugar and catecholamines.

5. Asafoetida (Hing)

Also known as

Latin	:	**Ferula foetida**
English	:	**Asafoetida**
Sanskrit	:	**Hingu**
Hindi	:	**Hing**
Marathi	:	**Hinga**
Tamil	:	**Perunkayanm**
Telugu	:	**Inguva**
Malayalam	:	**Kayam**
Kannada	:	**Hingu**

The Sanskrit word "Hingu" means "destroyer of cold and phlegm"

What is Hing—In the beginning of summer, the upper part of the root of a 4-5 year old plant is exposed and the stem cut off. This part is covered over by earth again and after a few days, the milky juice exuding from the cut surface is collected. The same procedure is repeated until the resin is exhausted. The dried resin is what we call asafoetida.

How it looks—It is a woody, perennial tree with huge, fleshy tapering roots.

What we use—Resinous exudate of the root

What it does—It is antispasmodic, carminative, digestive, expectorant, anthelmintic, emmenagogue and diuretic.

How we use it—

In **abdominal pain**—Warm a small piece of asafoetida in castor oil and mix well. This could be taken internally in adults and rubbed over the abdomen in infants and very small children. Asafoetida powder could be mixed in a glass of butter milk and taken too.

In **flatulence**—Fry a piece of asafoetida in some ghee and take ½ a tsp thrice a day to get relief from gaseous distension of abdomen.

In **indigestion**—Dissolve a couple of small pieces of asafoetida in half a cup of water and drink to relieve from gas, pain and for digestion.

As a preventive for fainting—Dissolve a piece of asafoetida in some lime juice and drink thrice a day to steer clear of fainting bouts.

In **dysmenorrhoea**—Use asafoetida fried in ghee regularly in diet to reduce the pain and discomfort accompanying menstrual periods and to promote free flow of fluid.

In **respiratory infections**—Take ½ a tsp of raw asafoetida twice a day before meals to clear the airways and reduce respiratory allergies.

In **urinary retention**—Fry asafoetida in ghee and take it washed down by some rice wash to promote flow of urine.

In **dental caries**—Heat asafoetida in a pan and fill the caried tooth with it.

Modern Study

Anti-microbial activity of essential oil extracted from the seed of Ferula foetida was demonstrated in experimental studies.

In **jaundice**—Dissolve a small part of asafoetida in water. Place it in both eyes twice a day.

In **hoarseness**—Take a small part of asafoetida with water twice a day.

In **opium poison**—Take asafoetida with water. It will neutralize the effect soon.

In **pinworm disease**—Take a small part of asafoetida in water. Place it in anus with the help of cotton. It will ease itching of anus.

Modern Study

Anti-microbial activity of essential oil extracted from the seed of Ferula foetida was demonstrated in experimental studies.

6. Ash Gourd (Petha)

Also known as

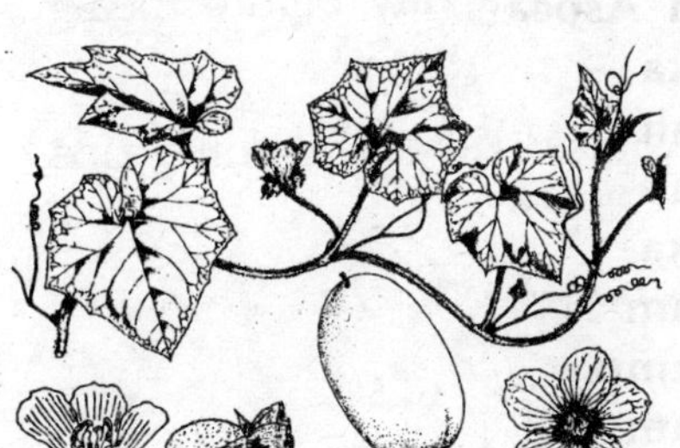

Latin	:	**Benincasa hispida**
English	:	**Ash Gourd, White Gourdmelon**
Sanskrit	:	**Kusmandah**
Hindi	:	**Petha, Raksa**
Marathi	:	**Kahala**
Tamil	:	**Pusanikkai**
Telugu	:	**Budidagummadi**
Malayalam	:	**Kumpalam**
Kannada	:	**Budikumbala**

How it looks—It is a large climbing gourd with large leaves, yellow flowers and broad cylindrical fruits.

What we use—Fruits, seeds

What it does—It is sweet, cooling, laxative, diuretic aphrodisiac and styptic

How we use it—

In **bleeding**—Whether internal or external, the intake of the juice of the ash pumpkin is highly helpful in arresting the bleeding and healing tissues.

In **excessive cholesterol**—It has been shown that regular intake of the juice of the ash pumpkin reduces cholesterol and dilates blood vessels.

In **sleeplessness**—The intake of the juice gives a feeling of satiation and induces sound sleep, so it can be used in disturbed or lack of sleep with impressive results.

In **burning urination**—In most urinary disorders regularly drinking the ash pumpkin juice increases the production of urine and even flushes out small urinary stones.

In **constipation**—Pieces of the fruit fried in ghee and the juice itself are laxative in nature.

In **worms**—About 20gms of the seeds are powdered and taken with honey on an empty stomach, followed by lots of the juice at night. The seeds being anthelmintic, this schedule usually frees the body from most intestinal worms.

In **anaemia**—The fruit and leaves are dried and powdered. A tsp of this powder is taken everyday with a glass of buttermilk.

As a brain tonic—The ash pumpkin is endowed with qualities such as nervine tonic and stimulant. A confectionery can be prepared with sugar candy, ghee, honey and the fruit pieces, which can be used in doses of a tsp everyday.

Modern Study

Ash pumpkin has been reported to be effective in the treatment of BPH (Benign Prostatic Hyperplasia or prostate enlargement).

7. Ashoka (Asoka)

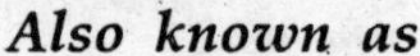

Also known as

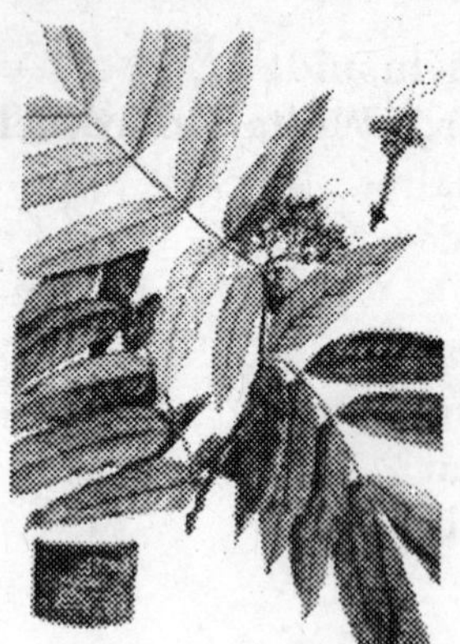

Latin : Saraca Asoca
English : Ashoka
Sanskrit : Asokah
Hindi : Asoka
Marathi : Ashoka
Tamil : Asokam
Telugu : Asokamu
Malayalam : Asokam
Kannada : Asokada

"Ashoka" in Sanskrit means "without distress"

How it looks—It is a medium-sized evergreen tree with spreading and drooping branches. It has orangish flowers which are fragrant. The fruits are flat, black pods with 4-8 seeds in each pod. The bark is dark brown to grey or black with an irregular surface, the cut ends of which are yellowish red in colour, turning reddish on exposure.

What we use—Bark, Leaves, flowers, seeds

What it does—*Bark*—astringent, sweet, refrigerant, anthelmintic styptic, demulcent, febrifuge

Flowers—uterine tonic

Leaves—depurative

How we use it—

In **uterine disorders**—It is a reputed uterine tonic especially useful in conditions of excessive or irregular bleeding, fibroids or white discharge.

Boil 2 tsp of the bark powder in 2 glasses of water until the water is reduced to a quarter of the quantity. Take an ounce of this filtered decoction twice a day with some honey to tone the mucosa of the uterus.

In **pimples**—To clear erupted skin, make a paste of Ashoka, some lime juice and milk and apply everyday.

In **piles**—Take a decoction of the bark mentioned above twice a day for relief from bleeding and non-bleeding piles.

In **abdominal pain**—Make a juice of the leaves, mix with cumin seeds and drink to relieve colicky pain in the abdomen.

In **burning sensation and inflammation**—The decoction of the bark can be used both internally as well as externally as a wash to relieve inflammation of any kind and to soothe burning sensation.

In **diabetes**—Powder the dry flowers of Ashoka and take a tsp of it everyday to keep blood sugar levels under control.

8. Babool (Babul)

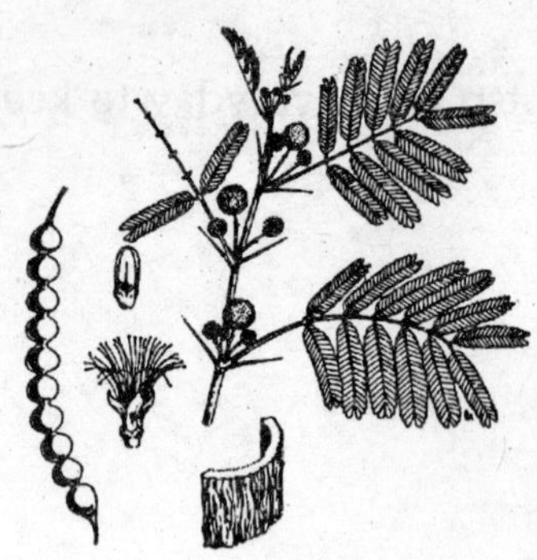

Also known as

Latin	:	**Acacia Arabica**
English	:	**Babool, Indian gum arabic tree**
Sanskrit	:	**Barburah**
Hindi	:	**Babul**
Marathi	:	**Babhula**
Tamil	:	**Karuvelam**
Telugu	:	**Nallatumma**
Malayalam	:	**Karivelam**
Kannada	:	**Karijali**

"That which binds stools" is the meaning of the Sanskrit word "Babbula"

How it looks—It is a moderate sized tree with dark brown or black, longitudinally fissured rough bark and reddish brown heartwood. The leaves are bipinnately compounds with glands on the main rachis. Straight, whitish sharp spines are present as stipules and flowers are golden yellow with rounded heads. The fruits are segmented pods holding 8-12 seeds each. The "gum arabic" exudes from cuts in the bark in ovoid globules and is coloured from pale yellow to black.

What we use—Bark, gum

What it does—*Bark* : Cooling, styptic, aphrodisiac, constipating, expectorant, emetic nutritive.

Gum—Cooling, emollient, expectorant, liver tonic, aphrodisiac, haemostatic, antipyretic, tonic.

How we use it—

In **diarrhoea**—Make a powder of the tender leaves of babool and take a tsp with water from time to time to correct stools.

In **wounds**—Sprinkle the powder of the tender leaves of babool over wounds for rapid healing.

In **excessive oozing from eyes**—Boil the decoction of the leaves of babool until it reaches a semi-solid consistency. Mix a tsp of this with honey and apply this like kajal to the inside of eyes to stop oozing.

In **fractures**—To help fractures heal better, take the powder of the fruits of babool, mix it with honey and take this for 3 days consecutively.

For **complexion of baby**—Chewing babool leaves during pregnancy enables a woman to deliver a baby with a clear, glowing complexion.

In **skin disorders**—Just like Khadira, the decoction of babool bark is also highly useful as a drink, bath water and to wash lesions. It mitigates burning sensation, restores normal colour to skin and heals ulcers and wounds quickly.

9. Bael (Bel)

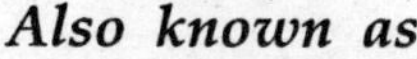

Also known as

Latin : Aegle marmelos
English : Bael tree, holy fruit tree
Sanskrit : Vilvah, sriphalah
Hindi : Bel
Marathi : Bela
Tamil : Kuvilam
Telugu : Bilwamu, Maredu
Malayalam : Kulakam
Kannada : Belapatri

How it looks—It is a medium-sized deciduous tree with typical straight sharp thorns at the axil and yellowish brown furrowed bark. The leaves are also notedly trifoliate and aromatic while the flowers are greenish white and sweet scented. The fruits are globose and woody with yellowish rind with numerous seeds.

What we use—Roots, leaves, fruits (usually unripe ones are used)

What it does—*Roots*—Astringent, febrifuge

Leaves—Astringent, laxative, febrifuge, expectorant

Unripe fruits—Astringent, digestive stomachic

Ripe fruits—Astringent, aromatic, cooling, febrifuge, laxative and tonic (to the heart & brain)

How we use it—

In **piles**—Make a decoction of the roots of Bael and seat the piles' patient in a basin filled with the lukewarm decoction such that the pile masses are immersed in it. Do this everyday for 20-30 minutes and watch the astringent Bael gradually shrink the pile masses.

In **dysentery and diarrhoea**—Paste the pulp of an unripe bael fruit with a few sesame seeds and mix some thick yogurt in it. Take this preparation twice a day to arrest mucous and blood-accompanied loose stools.

In **blood-accompanied stools**—Mix the powder of the dry pulp of bael fruit with some saunph seeds and honey and drink 2 tsp of this mixture with some rice wash.

In **foul body odour**—Apply the juice of the fresh leaves of bael fruit all over the body everyday to prevent unpleasant odour emitting from the body. The astringent nature of the juice closes sweat pores and prevents excessive perspiration causing foul odour.

In **vomiting**—Make a decoction of bael roots and drink it with a tsp of honey to suppress vomiting.

In **bleeding piles**—Mix the pulp of a bael fruit with a glass of butter milk for relief from bleeding piles.

In **swelling**—Whether of the feet or any part of body, swellings can be helped by taking half a glass of the juice of bael leaves with the powder of a few black peppers.

In **colic pains**—In pains due to undigested food material, take the powder of the dry pulp of bael fruit with a little jaggery for digestion and to subside pain.

In **typhoid and seasonal fevers**—Take a tsp of powder of the dry pulp of bael fruit to bring down temperature.

In **decomposing wounds**—Paste the leaves without adding water. Apply this on wounds which are pus-oozing with great benefit.

10. Bamboo (Bans)

Also known as

Latin	:	**Bambusa arundinacea**
English	:	**Bamboo**
Sanskrit	:	**Vamsah**
Hindi	:	**Bans**
Marathi	:	**Velu**
Tamil	:	**Mulmunkil**
Telugu	:	**Vedurubiyyam**
Malayalam	:	**Mula, Illi**
Kannada	:	**Bedru**

How it looks—It is a tall thorny shrub with many stems held on a stout root stock. The stem sheath is orange-yellow and streaked. The leaf sheaths are short, bristly and often occupy the whole stem. Flowers are glumes and fruits are oblong grains.

What we use—Roots leaves, sprouts, grains, and bamboo manna.

What it does—*Roots*—Cooling, laxative, diuretic tonic

Leaves—Cooling emmenagogue, vulnerary, febrifuge, constrictive

Sprouts—Laxative, thermogenic, anti-inflammatory, digestive, carminative, anthelmentic and diuretic.

Grains—Anthelmentic, aphrodisiac, tonic

Bamboo manna—It is the siliceous secretion found in the internodes of the stems. It occurs as a bluish white translucent mass. This dried sugar-like granules are called bamboo manna. It is expectorant, haemostatic, aphrodisiac, diuretic, febrifuge.

How we use it—

In **mouth ulcers**—Apply pasted bamboo manna on the ulcers to effect a quick cure.

In **piles**—Make a decoction of the leaves of bamboo and pour it into a shallow tub. Seat the piles patient in this tub so that the pile masses are completely immersed in the decoction. Do this every day for 15 minutes for shrinkage of pile masses.

In **eye inflammations**—Paste the roots of bamboo in water and instill a few drops in the eyes to prevent infections and cure inflammation at early stages.

In **bleeding disorders**—Paste bamboo manna pieces with some saumph seeds and take everyday until bleeding is controlled.

In **worm infestation**—Dissolve pieces of bamboo manna in water and add a few crushed cumin seeds to it. This preparation taken internally dislodges worms and expels them.

In **cough & other respiratory disorders**—Soothing to the throat and expectorant ,manna is highly useful in coughs of all kinds. Powdered manna with some honey is ideal to lick down in such conditions. It has soothing activity on lung tissue.

In **diarrhoea and dysentery**—The organic salts present in bamboo ensure improvement in the quality of blood, and even bone and elastic tissue. This is why it works effectively in bleeding and its astringent and digestive properties make it a good anti-diarrhoeal.

In **scanty urination**—Bamboo also has gentle action on the urinary tissue and is therefore used dissolved in water as a diuretic.

In **consumption and wasting diseases**—Rubbed with amla fruit and honey, it makes a preparation called "Murabba" which is highly nutritive and aphrodisiac.

11. Banana (Kela)

Also known as

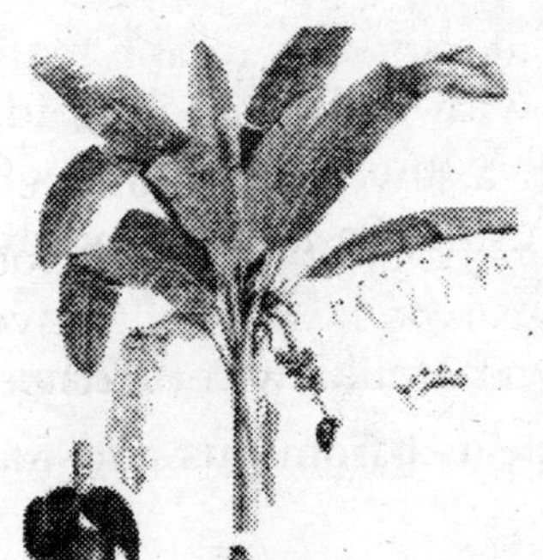

Latin	:	Musa sapientum
English	:	Banana
Sanskrit	:	Kadali
Hindi	:	Kela
Marathi	:	Kela/Keli
Tamil	:	Kadali
Telugu	:	Ariti
Malayalam	:	Kadalivala
Kannada	:	Valchannu

The very botanical name of banana, Musa paradisiaca, "Apple of paradise" suggests that it is one of the oldest fruits in the world.

Originating from the east of India and neighboring countries, it has gained popularity over centuries and has been taken to America, Africa, Palestine and Egypt by invaders and visitors making it commercially the most important tropical fruit now.

Often called the most delicious thing in the world, the seedless fruit has gained the status of the staple food of millions around the world, so much so that the soft ripe banana is the first solid food given to babies.

Vitamins—The ripe fruit is a rich source of Vit-A and a moderate source of vitamins C,B and B_2.

The unripe fruit is an excellent source of vitamins which do not perish even after cooking at temperatures upto 60°C

Minerals—Magnesium, potassium and phosphorus are some of the minerals present abundantly in the fruit and calcium and iron are others moderately found in it.

Sugar—The numerous varieties of banana contain glucose levels varying between 15 and 27 percent.

Fibre—The stem is rich in fibre and is cooked as a curry in banana – growing regions. Even the inflorescence is made into a curry in the north-eastern regions.

Strictly speaking, the term plantain is used for the cooking variety of banana, though now, both terms are used intermixed.

How it looks—It is a fleshy, decorative tall herb with long sheathing leaves and bright yellow fruits (on ripening)

What we use—Root, leaves, fruit, stem

What it does—*Roots*—anthelmintic, antiscorbutic, depurative and tonic

Fruits—sweet, astringent, emollient, aphrodisiac, anthelmintic antidiabetic, antidysenteric

How we use it—

In **urinary retention**—Take a glassful of the stem juice with a few cardamom seeds crushed into it thrice a day to get rid of painful or burning urination and to dissolve tiny urinary stones.

In **anaemia**—Take a tsp of the powder of the dried root with milk twice a day.

In **wounds**—Tie the ripe, clean leaves onto the wounds, to clear it from pus and foul odour. Change this dressing twice a day.

In **white discharge**—One of the best remedies for excessive vaginal discharge is to mix a tsp of the powder of dried amla seeds and a ripe banana everyday for at least 40 days.

In **constipation**—A ripe banana with hot milk at bedtime every night is a well known smooth laxative for hard bowels.

In **menorrhagia** or any other **bleeding condition**—The fruit of plantain should be consumed everyday mixed with ghee to arrest bleeding either from rectum due to piles, excessive menstrual bleeding, or any other internal bleeding.

In **cough and breathing disorders**—Roast a banana and peel it after cooling. The banana, so baked should be consumed everyday to relieve from respiratory distress.

When hair is swallowed—Make a curry of plantain stem and consume. The roughage present in it rolls into its bulk hair and other matter present in the alimentary canal and eliminates them.

In **boils**—Scrape the inside of a ripe banana peel, spread it on a cloth and bandage on to the boil to effect quick healing.

In **burns**—In an emergency, when nothing is available a banana comes in handy. Mash a yellow ripe banana and spread it over the burn. The demulcent effect of the fruit quickens healing and prevents scar formation. Repeat this procedure for a few days.

In **fungal infections**—Mix the yellow ripe banana in neem decoction and apply on the patches and wash after half an hour. Repeat until cure is effected.

As a **cosmetic**—The fruit pulp is mixed in honey or used as such as a face mask.

Modern Study

Experimental studies on Musa paradisiaca (banana) in Brazil, showed antiulcer effects in all the models studied.

Bananas are highly nutritious and are essential in the diet of the pregnant and lactating woman, growing children and the aged.

12. Banyan (Bat)

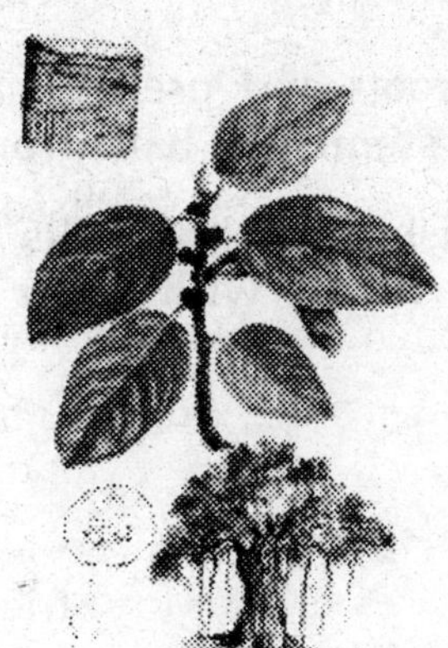

Also known as

Latin	:	Ficus benghalensis
English	:	Banyan tree
Sanskrit	:	Nyagrodhah
Hindi	:	Bat, Baragad
Marathi	:	Vata
Tamil	:	Alamaram
Telugu	:	Peddamarri
Malayalam	:	Peral
Kannada	:	Ala

How it looks—It is a very large tree with widely spreading branches having typical aerial roots-prop roots. The bark is greenish white and the fruit, contained in red, fleshy receptacles.

What we use—Aerial root, bark, leaves, buds, fruit, latex.

What it does—Astringent, refrigerant, anodyne, depurative, anti-inflammatory, styptic, antiarthritic, antidiarrhoeal, anti-emetic, tonic.

How we use it—

In **sterility in women**—Powder the dry roots finely and store. Take a tsp of this powder with half a glass of cow's milk at bedtime, for at least 3 menstrual cycles.

In **white discharge and vomiting**—Make a decoction of the aerial roots and consume half a glass twice a day.

In **skin disorders**—Whether it is burning sensation, scars, abscesses or ulcers, the banyan has an answer. Paste banyan and peepal bark in coconut milk and apply on the affected areas to prevent scars and heal ulcers.

In **diarrhoea and dysentery**—Soak the buds of the banyan tree in water overnight and take the infusion every morning until diarrhoea is controlled.

In **bleeding piles**—Mix a few drops of the milky latex of the banyan tree in milk and take daily to cure bleeding piles.

In **painful joints**—The milky juice from the banyan tree is good to massage aching joints with, as it relieves swelling and rheumatic pain.

Tooth care—The aerial roots of the banyan make for effective toothbrushes, owing to the astringent secretions from the stick which is to be chewed while brushing.

Hair growth—Powder equal quantities of the aerial roots of banyan and lime skin. Boil the powder in coconut oil and store. This oil promotes hair growth and leaves hair with a fine sheen.

In baldness—Powder the aerial roots of banyan and lotus roots and use the same way as above. This preparation irritates the bald scalp and stimulates hair growth.

In sex—To improve sexual activity, eating fruits is an established treatment. Its fruit is collected and dried in shade. Then it is powdered and mixed with sugar (for taste) and taken three times a day with water.

13. Betel Nut (Supari)

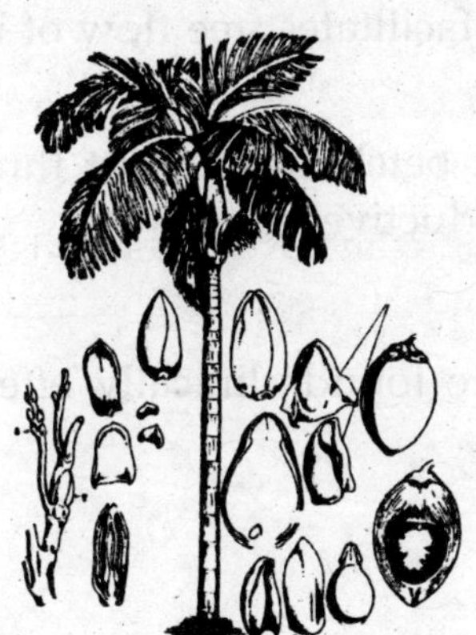

Also known as

Latin	:	**Areca Catechu**
English	:	**Betel nut, arecanut**
Sanskrit	:	**Pugah**
Hindi	:	**Supari**
Marathi	:	**Supari**
Tamil	:	**Pakkumaram**
Telugu	:	**Vakka**
Malayalam	:	**Kavennu**
Kannada	:	**Adike**

How it looks—It is a slender unbranched palm with a crown of pinnate leaves and a ringed stem. The flowers are in a spadix and fruits are smooth and reddish or orange when ripe.

What we use—Roots, leaves, fruits

What it does—It is cooling, astringent, diuretic, digestive, anthelmintic, aphrodisiac, nervine tonic, emmenagogue and antibacterial.

How we use it—

In **sore lips**—Take a decoction of the root as a cure for cracked and sore lips. Its cooling and astringent properties ensure quick healing.

In **back pain**—Juice the tender leaves and mix with oil. Use this emulsion as a pack for the lower back with a piece of cloth and leave on for 20 minutes. You will notice the pain seeping away.

In **worm infestation**—The cured arecanuts should be ground in buttermilk and the paste should be eaten to cure worm infestation-especially tapeworm.

As a **digestive**—The cured nuts are pounded and mixed with mouth fresheners and digestives like edible camphor, cardamom and poppy seeds, to make the market- available betel nut powder. Usually chewed after a meal, it clears the mouth and stomach, gives a sense of satiation and helps in digesting even the heaviest of meals.

Tooth care—Chewing the boiled (cured) nuts promotes salivation and thereby helps heal ulcers apart from preventing tooth decay. Still, it must be remembered that its constant use blackens teeth and loosens them.

The charred powder of the nut has always been in vogue as an effective tooth powder for cleansing and strengthening teeth.

In constipation :The juice of the tender nuts is laxative in nature and can be given in mild constipation at bed time.

In **dysuria**—Water boiled with the areca nut is diuretic and facilitates free flow of urine apart from being a coolant to the body.

In **cough**—Betel nuts chewed along with the leaves of the betel climber, cut through phlegm and expectorate it and thereby are useful in productive cough.

Modern Study

Areca catechu was an important ingredient of a toothpaste found clinically effective in controlling dental diseases in a study in Udaipur.

14. Betel (Pan)

Also known as

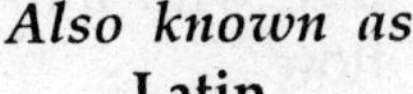

Latin	:	**Piper betle**
English	:	**Betel**
Sanskrit	:	**Thambulavalli**
Hindi	:	**Pan, Tambuli**
Marathi	:	**Nagveli**
Tamil	:	**Vathalaikkodi**
Telugu	:	**Thamalapaku**
Malayalam	:	**Vetulakkoli**
Kannada	:	**Vilyadele**

How it looks—It is a perennial climber, with semi-woody stem. The leaves are heart-shaped resembling pepper leaves and are bright green in colour. Fruits are rarely produced, immersed in fleshy spikes forming nodule- like structures.

What we use—Whole plant

What it does—It is astringent, carminative, stomachic, sialogogue, anthelmentic, aromatic, aphrodisiac, expectorant, febrifuge, laxative and tonic.

How we use it—

In **filariasis**—Take 7 betel leaves and paste them with a little sendha or rock salt. Take it with warm water everyday for a few weeks in filariasis.

In **worm infestation**—In such a common ailment, chewing pan leaves and spitting the juice out serves to remove immature larvae from the mouth reducing intensity of infection

In **phlegmatic cough and cold**—Chewing betel leaves is highly beneficial as it is an expectorant and helps break down solidified phlegm and expel it.

You could also combine the juices of the leaves of tulsi, betel and karpuravalli or panjiri-ka-pat. A few drops of the mixture with a tsp of honey is the safest and best remedy for cough in small children.

In **ulcerated burns**—Bathe the burns in betel leaf juice. The astringent action of betel helps regenerate cells and quickens healing.

In **fungal infections**—Especially over the face, back and chest, applying a mixture of onion and betel juice twice a day ensures getting rid of patches immediately.

In **headache**—A simple home remedy is to cut a betel leaf into 2 halves lengthwise, gently warm the halves over fire and apply over each temple. Its aromatic and tonic properties help soothe the headache.

In **difficult urination**—Mix betel leaf juice with milk, add some sugar and drink it to promote urination and ensure free flow.

In **whitlow**—To heal this finger infection, make a paste of quicklime and betel, pack the finger with this and tie a cloth around it. Change the pack everyday and keep the finger free of moisture. Cure is usually complete in 4-5 days.

In **fresh eye inflammation**—Instill a few drops of a mixture of betel leaf juice and honey to combat infection and effect quick healing.

15. Bitter Gourd (Karela)

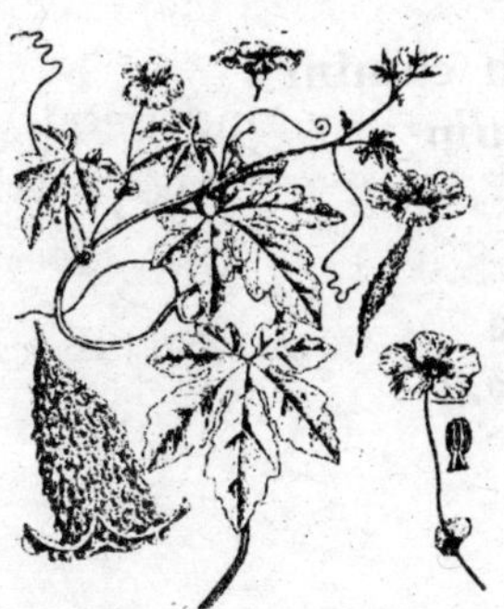

Also known as

Latin	:	**Momordica charantia**
English	:	**Bitter Gourd, Carillafruit**
Sanskrit	:	**Karavelaka**
Hindi	:	**Karela**
Marathi	:	**Karale**
Tamil	:	**Pavakkay**
Telugu	:	**Kakara**
Malayalam	:	**Kaypa**
Kannada	:	**Hagalakayi**

How it looks—It is a branching climber with angled stems, beaked and ribbed fruits and shining even seeds.

What we use—Whole plant

What it does—*Roots*—Astringent

Leaves—Anthelmintic, emetic and purgative

Fruits—Purgative, antidiabetic, emmenagogue, anti-inflammatory

How we use it—

In **gout**—The oil prepared from the decoction of the leaves of bittergourd makes a soothing topical application in gout.

In **cholera**—Drink the juice of bitter gourd with some sesame oil twice a day to arrest the vomiting and diarrhoea associated with cholera.

In **worm infestations**—Paste the leaves of bittergourd, roll them into balls and consume 1-2 balls for a good deworming.

In **burning sensation of hands and feet**—The juice of bittergourd leaves should be applied topically to alleivate the burning sensation.

In **delayed periods**—Taking a decoction of the roots of bitter gourd at least twice a day usually makes the period commence.

As a **diet**—

In **fevers and swellings**—The entire plant may be used in various preparations like curry, soup, or vegetable, to reduce swelling and bring down temperature.

In **measles**—The juice of the leaves of bitter gourd with turmeric serves as a cleansing drink during an attack of measles.

In **diabetes**—Probably the most celebrated use of the bittergourd in diseases is in checking blood sugar levels in diabetes. A glass of the juice or decoction of the leaves every morning on empty stomach along with a balanced diet is effective in keeping diabetes under control.

16. Black Plum (Jamun)

Also known as

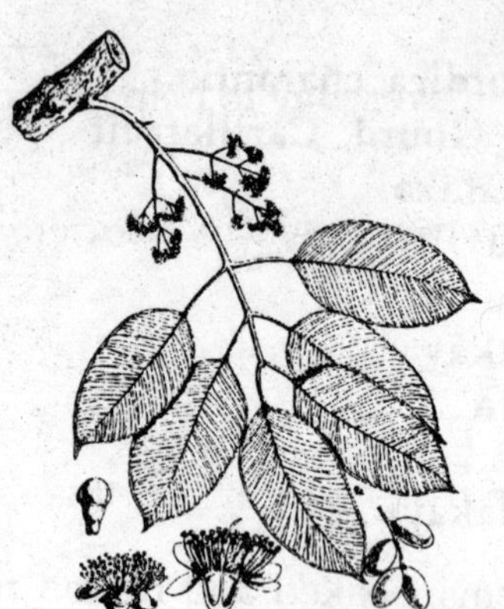

Latin	:	Syzigium cumini
English	:	Black plum
Sanskrit	:	Jambuh
Hindi	:	Jamun
Marathi	:	Jambhula
Tamil	:	Kottainaval
Telugu	:	Neredu
Malayalam	:	Naval
Kannada	:	Nerale

How it looks—It is a medium sized tree usually cultivated in the roads for shade with a smooth light grey bark with dark patches and greenish white flowers. The fruits are dark purple and oblong with pink pulp and a single seed in each.

What we use—Bark, fruits and leaves.

What it does—*Bark*—astringent, refrigerant, carminative, diuretic, digestive, anthelmintic, constipating

Leaves—antibacterial

Fruits/seeds—tonic, cooling

How we use it—

In **diarrhoea and dysentery**—Dried and powdered jamun seeds are mixed with mango seed powder and jaggery. A small roll of this mixture should be taken thrice a day to arrest diarrhoea.

Alternately, the powder of the bark should be mixed in milk and honey and consumed twice a day.

In **vomiting due to hyperacidity**—The cooled decoction of the tender leaves of mango and jamun is mixed with a little honey and taken twice a day for relief from vomiting and burning sensation.

In **wounds**—The fine powder of the bark is sprinkled on the fresh wound for quick healing and to arrest bleeding.

In **bleeding from any orifice**—The decoction of the bark powder is cooled and mixed with honey before drinking to arrest the bleeding.

In **white discharge**- Paste jamun roots in water in which rice has been washed and take it twice a day with the same.

In **diabetes**—Dried jamun fruit should be powdered with the seeds and a tsp of this powder is taken twice a day to prevent the loss of glucose in urine. The fruit can also generally be included in the diet of a diabetic.

In **enlargement of spleen**—Take an ounce of the juice of jamun everyday to help improve the general health in this condition.

In **difficult micturition**—Drink the diluted juice of jamun frequently to increase production of urine and relieve this condition.

In **pus-filled wounds**—The paste of the leaves serves as a good poultice to drain pus-filled abscesses.

In **indigestion**—The jamun fruit is a very powerful digestive and can be taken in conditions where even hair has been swallowed.

Modern Studies

1. Experimental studies on jamun seed extract showed decrease in aggressive behaviour, and analgesic activity in rats.
2. Jamun was found to be one of the effective food supplements in cases of non-insulin dependent diabetes mellitus.

17. Camphor (Kapur)

Also known as

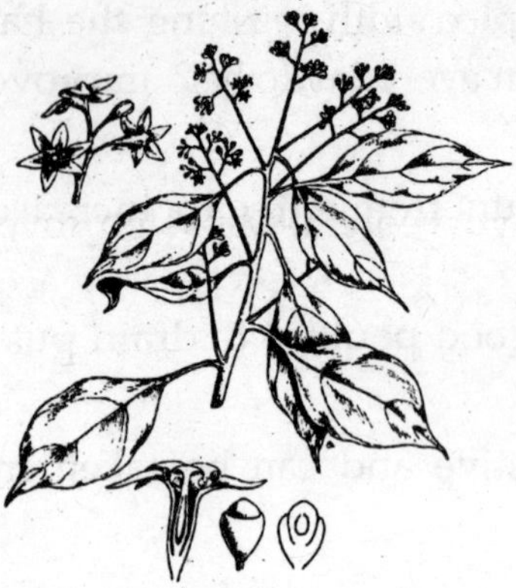

Latin	:	Cinnamomum camphora
English	:	Camphor tree
Sanskrit	:	Karpurah
Hindi	:	Kapur
Marathi	:	Kapura
Tamil	:	Karpuram
Telugu	:	Paccakarpuram
Malayalam	:	Cutakrpuram
Kannada	:	Karpura

How it looks—An attractive, thickly branched evergreen tall tree, it is adorned by yellowish-white flowers and bears dark green fruits which turn dark brown on ripening.

Camphor is the oil distilled mainly from the cells of the leaves and stem.

What we use—Deposits in the oil cells (camphor)

What it does—It is aromatic, skin and cardiac stimulant, antiseptic, aphrodisiac and expectorant.

How we use it—

In **wounds**—Camphor is powdered, pasted in ghee and applied over the affected area to relieve pain and inflammation.

In **joint pains**—Heat sesame oil, remove from stove and add a few pieces of camphor to make an effective application on painful joints. In cold places, mustard oil may be used instead of sesame oil.

In **muscle cramps**—An ointment can be made of camphor and sesame oil and applied to relieve from cramps.

In **toothaches**—Hold a piece of cotton soaked in camphor oil between teeth to numb ache, or you could press camphor and pepper powder on the tooth.

In **common cold**—It is used as a smelling salt in bouts of cold. Put a few drops on a hanky and sniff to clear stuffy nose.

In **burning sensation**—Powdered camphor is dissolved in bath water. Sandal pastes may be added to enhance the effect.

In **burns**—Powdered camphor in oil make a highly healing application over burns.

In **itching around the anus**—Make a paste of thymol and camphor, or camphor and just sesame oil to make a soothing ointment.

In **itching eczema**—Camphor can be added to any preparation for healing an itchy lesion, as it numbs and thereby soothes the urge to scratch.

In **lice infestation**—Adding camphor to coconut oil , coupled with washing the hair with dilute camphor for water keeps lice at bay.

Modern Study

Camphor was found to be an important ingredient of an Ayurvedic toothpaste proved clinically effective in curing dental disorders.

18. Cardamom (Elaichi)

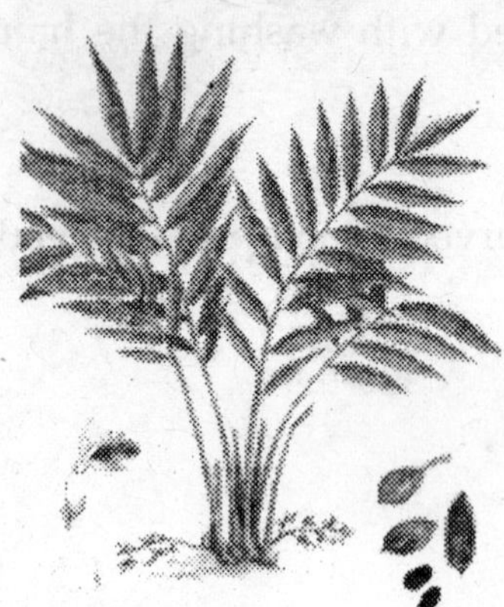

Also known as

Latin	:	Elettaria Cardamom
English	:	Cardamom
Sanskrit	:	Ela
Hindi	:	Elaichi
Marathi	:	Velachi
Tamil	:	Elam
Telugu	:	Elakkayalu
Malayalam	:	Elam
Kannada	:	Elakki

How it looks—It is a tall perennial herb with a branching root stock under the ground. The sharp-edged leaves have a sheathing base. The flowers and fruits arise from the base of the stem near the ground, the fruits being three-sided with many black, fragrant seeds.

What we use—Seeds, oil

What it does—*Seeds*—aromatic, cooling, stimulant, digestive, carminative, stomachic diuretic, cardiotonic, expectorant, abortifacient and tonic.

How we use it—

In **vomiting**—Boil a cardamom fruit and some ginger pieces in a glass of water and allow to cool. Take this water in doses of an ounce thrice a day to drive away nausea and vomiting.

To **stimulate appetite**—Add a few cardamom seeds and some ginger pieces to your tea as an appetiser and to improve taste perception.

In **headache**—Paste the skin of a large cardamom and apply it to the forehead. You can also add a clove and the stalk of a betel leaf to this application

In **thirst/hiccups**—Boil a few cardamom seeds in a glass of water and drink to quench long standing thirst especially due to a fatty meal. The same water can be used for relief from hiccups too.

In **flatulence**—To relieve discomfort due to gaseous distension of the abdomen, just chew a few cardamoms.

In **urinary disorders**—For an excellent diuretic, mix a tsp of cardamom seed powder and amla juice and drink twice a day.

In **heart disorders**—In Ayurvedic classics, cardamom is held to be an excellent cardiac tonic. You could paste the roots of cardamom with some ghee and take everyday to tone your heart.

In **throat irritation**—Chewing on cardamom soothes the throat and clears any obstructing phlegm.

Modern Study

Anti-inflammatory activity of the essential oil of cardamom was found in experimental studies on rats.

In experimental studies on mice, the oil exhibited analgesic properties.

19. Carrot (Gajar)

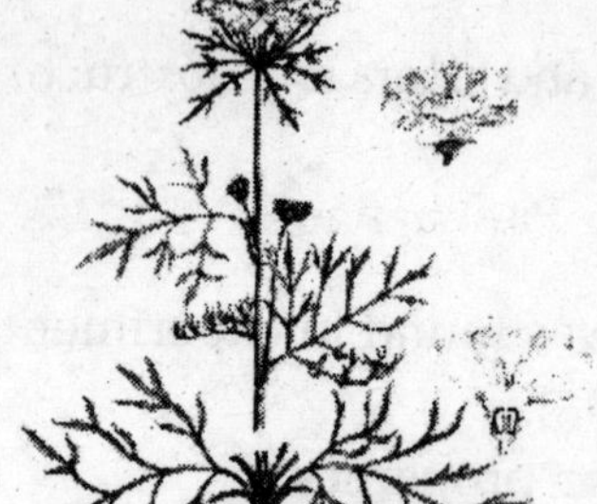

Also known as

Latin	**:**	**Daucas Carota**
English	**:**	**Carrot, Bee's nest**
Sanskrit	**:**	**Garjarah**
Hindi	**:**	**Gajar**
Marathi	**:**	**Gajar**
Tamil	**:**	**Gajjarakkilangu**
Telugu	**:**	**Gajjaragadda**
Malayalam	**:**	**Karattu**
Kannada	**:**	**Gajjari**

How it looks—It is a biennial herb with a branched erect stem and a yellow conical tap root. The leaves are thin and decompound and flowers small, white or yellowish. The fruits are long with bristly hairs.

What we use—Roots, seeds.

What it does—*Tap roots*—sweet, thermogenic, appetiser, digestive, anthelmintic, aphrodisiac, cardiotonic, expectorant.

Seeds—aromatic, stimulant, aphrodisiac, diuretic, abortifacient.

How we use it—

To **improve complexion**—Drinking white radish and carrot juice at least twice a week to ensure a blemish-free complexion. They contain Vit-A and also act as diuretics flushing out toxins from the system.

In **kidney disease**—Carrot seeds should be made into a decoction and used every day to reduce swelling.

In **excessive internal heat**—Fresh carrot juice should be used regularly to revive the run-down system.

In **eye trouble**—Take the juice of fresh root in a cup. Mix it with 250gm of fennel and 10gm of sugar. Take this mixture with milk before going to bed.

In **dysentery**—Boil the roots and extract juice. Take juice one cup thrice a day.

20. Castor (Erand)

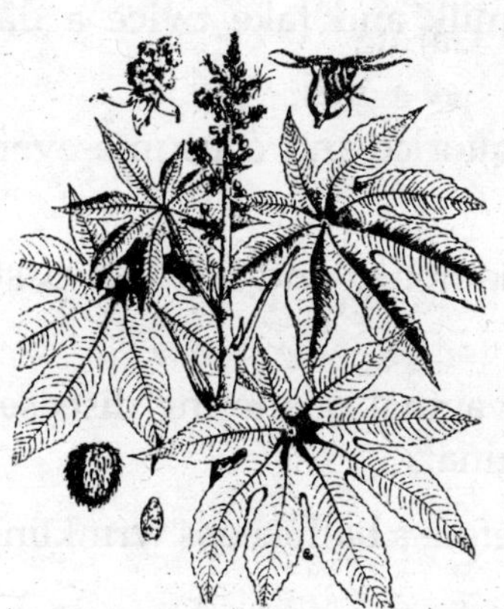

Also known as

Latin	:	**Ricinus communis**
English	:	**Castor**
Sanskrit	:	**Erandah, Panchangula**
Hindi	:	**Erand**
Marathi	:	**Enanda**
Tamil	:	**Amanakku**
Telugu	:	**Amudamu**
Malayalam	:	**Avanakku**
Kannada	:	**Haralu**

How it looks—It is a bushy, small tree with thin greyish brown bark, typical palmate leaves with conspicuous glands. The green fruits are covered with fresh prickles (when young) enclosing oil-bearing seeds.

What we use—Roots, leaves, flowers, seed oil

What it does—*Roots*— aphrodisiac, purgative, carminative, anthelmintic, galactogogue, expectorant

Leaves—diuretic, anthelmintic, galactogogue

Seeds—digestive, aphrodisiac

Seed oil—antipyretic, thermogenic

How we use it—

In **ascitis and amoebiasis**—Milk boiled with the root powder of castor should be taken every night for regularising bowel movements and to stop blood and pus from being passed along with stools.

In **gout and hernia**—The seeds of castor are crushed in milk and consumed twice a day to relieve from gouty pains. A diet of rice is beneficial while following this remedy. In hernia, this treatment should be followed for a month.

In **eye care**—Instilling a few drops of castor oil in the eyes before retiring to bed is an excellent practice for long eyelashes, lustrous eyes and good vision. In night blindness chewing the leaves of castor is helpful in improving eyesight.

In **piles**—Boil castor leaves in water and steadily pour the lukewarm water on pile masses to reduce pain and the pile masses themselves.

Drink a decoction of triphala (harad, amla and vibheetaki) mixed with 1 tsp of castor oil to relieve constipation and soften pile masses.

As an **aphrodisiac**—The roots of castor taken in any form such as decoction, paste or juice, increase libido and enhance sexual performance.

In **sciatica and back pain**—Crush the seeds of castor in milk and take twice a day to lubricate joints and relieve pain in any form.

In **colicky pain**—Add a little castor oil to a decoction of liquorice and consume every 3 hours to subside pain.

In **jaundice**—Mix a tsp of the root powder of castor in some honey and lick this paste twice a day to cleanse the system.

As a **vaginal douche**—In pain during intercourse, or any vaginal or uterine diseases, soak a piece of cotton in castor oil and place in the vagina.

As a **cosmetic**—Smearing castor oil over the body and head before a bath keeps wrinkling, greying of hair and balding at bay.

21. Chebulic Myrobylan (Harad)

Also known as

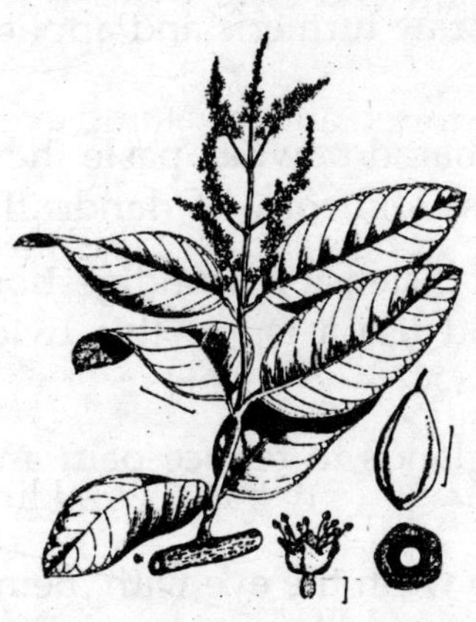

Latin	:	Terminalia chebula
English	:	Chebulic myrobylan
Sanskrit	:	Haritaki, Pathya, Abhaya
Hindi	:	Harad
Marathi	:	Hirada
Tamil	:	Katukkay
Telugu	:	Karakkaya
Malayalam	:	Katukka
Kannada	:	Harra

How it looks—It is a moderate to large, deciduous tree with a rounded crown, spreading branches and yellowish white flowers. The shiny ovoid fruits are yellow to orange brown in colour with hard, pale yellow seeds.

What we use—*Mature and immature fruits.*

What it does—It is astringent, thermogenic, anodyne, anti-inflammatory, stomachic, laxative, purgative, digestive, carminative, anthelmintic, aphrodisiac, diuretic and febrifuge.

How we use it—

In **piles**—Taking a tsp of harad powder with jaggery before food is highly beneficial due to its astringent and laxative properties.

In **hiccough**—Powder of harad with hot water in a dose of 5gm thrice a day relieves even long-standing hiccoughs.

In **vomiting**—Licking the powder of harad with honey is a sure remedy for nausea and vomiting.

In **throat infections**—1 tsp of honey should be mixed in a glass of decoction of harad and consumed, twice a day.

In **bleeding disorders & hyperacidity**—Take equal quantities of harad powder and raisins, to your liking. Over a period of time you will find the bleeding corrected and hyperacidity relieved.

In **arthritis**—Mix a tsp of harad powder in castor oil and swallow. This relieves the pain and swelling and smoothens joint movements.

In **low appetite**—½ tsp each of sonth powder, jaggery, harad powder and sendha powder should be eaten daily before meals.

In **excessive perspiration**—Rub a fine powder of harad all over body. Wait for a few minutes and rinse off with a bath.

In **whitlow**—Harad powder should be ground in the juice of raw turmeric and applied on the affected finger nail.

In **dandruff**—Powder the kernel of mango fruit, mix it with harad powder, paste them in milk and apply on scalp regularly to vanquish the most stubborn of dandruff.

In **abdominal pain**—Pain in the abdomen may be due to gas distension or indigestion. Grind harad, nutmeg and sweet flag or bach to a paste and use a tsp of this twice a day.

In **mumps**—Apply a thick paste of harad on the inflamed glands to reduce pain and swelling.

In **eye inflammation**—Cool and filter a decoction of harad to wash the eye with. Being astringent and healing, it relieves the swelling and redness quickly.

In **toothache**—Apply a fine powder of harad directly on the painful tooth for relief from the ache.

In **fungal infections and scabies**—Apply a paste of harad and turmeric to the affected part twice a day until the skin turns completely normal.

In any **skin allergy**—Wash the area with harad decoction and drink the same twice a day.

In **obesity**—Use triphala powder – a combination of "harad,bahera and amla" (chebulic and belleric myrobylan and gooseberry) a tsp daily with honey on empty stomach and watch the fat melt away after a couple of months.

Modern Study

Harad was an important ingredient of an ayurvedic tooth paste found effective against dental diseases.

22. Chirata (Cirayata)

Also known as

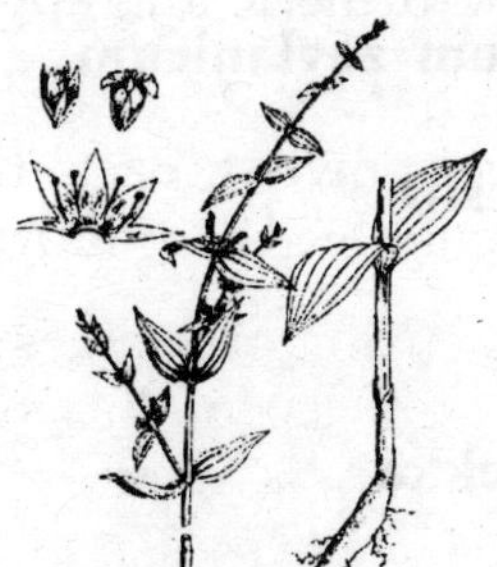

Latin	**:**	**Swertia chirayita**
English	**:**	**Chirata**
Sanskrit	**:**	**Kiratatikta**
Hindi	**:**	**Cirayata**
Marathi	**:**	**Kadechirayit**
Tamil	**:**	**Cirattakucci**
Telugu	**:**	**Nelavemu**
Malayalam	**:**	**Uttarakiriyattu**
Kannada	**:**	**Nelabevu**

How it looks—It is an erect annual herb, with strong stems which are cylindrical below and four-angled towards the top. The leaves are lance-shaped with 5 nerves along the length and the flowers are many, small and greenish yellow. The fruits are minute, pointed, capsules with smooth many-angled seeds.

What we use—Whole plant

What it does—It is both refrigerant and thermogenic, anti-inflammatory, antipyretic, sudorific and anti periodic.

How we use it—

In **fevers**—In fevers of all types, chirata is highly useful either singly or in combination with other herbs like picrohiza, tinospora, bittergourd or snakegourd. Make a decoction of chirata and drink thrice a day to conquer even obstinate and chronic fevers.

In **worms**—Give a decoction of the leaves sweetened with palm candy to children afflicted with worms at bed time.

In **skin disease**—Pasted with oil and a few pepper seeds and applied on itchy patches, chirata purifies blood and heals and soothes rashes and irritation. Intake of chirata berries is preventive for skin disease.

In **swellings**—Powder the dried plant of chirata and dry ginger and take a tsp of powder with some rice wash twice a day to reduce swelling of feet, hands or face.

In **bleeding disorders**—Take half a tsp each of the powders of chirata and sandal with cool water thrice a day especially to control excessive bleeding.

To **purify breast milk**—To keep breast milk free of infections and to promote secretion and flow of milk, drink a decoction of chirata everyday for a week.

In **mouth ulcers**—Soak the berries in buttermilk overnight and then dry and powder them for storage. Whenever necessary, fry a tsp of this powder in ghee and mix with rice before eating to soothe oral ulcers.

23. Cinnamon (Dalchini)

Also known as

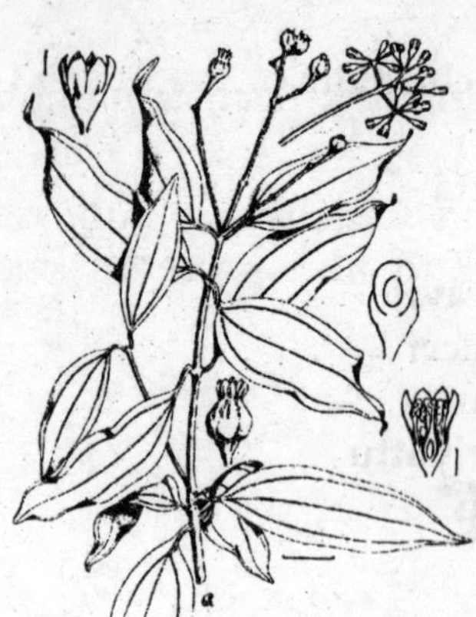

Latin	**:**	**Cinnamomum zeylanicum**
English	**:**	**Cinnamon**
Sanskrit	**:**	**Tvak, Darusita**
Hindi	**:**	**Dalchini**
Marathi	**:**	**Dalchini**
Tamil	**:**	**Elavangam**
Telugu	**:**	**Dalchinichekka**
Malayalam	**:**	**Elavangam**
Kannada	**:**	**Dalchini**

How it looks—It is a moderate sized evergreen tree with reddish brown soft bark, with warts and dark purple ovoid fruits.

What we use—Bark, oil

What it does—Bark—Acrid, aromatic, astringent, aphrodisiac, febrifuge, diuretic, carminative.

How we use it—

In **dysentery**—Half a tsp of the powder of the leaves is taken everyday to control dysentery.

In **headache**—Rub the oil lightly onto the temples to ward off headaches.

In **vomiting**—Add a few drops of the oil to water/milk and drink for nausea and vomiting to subside.

In **heavy periods**—Take a glass of the decoction of the bark twice a day to control heavy menstrual bleeding.

In **cavities in teeth**—A piece of cotton soaked in the oil held in between teeth helps keep infection away.

In **wheezing**—Boil pieces of cinnamon, liquorice and palm candy in 3 cups of water and reduce to a cup. Take an ounce of this decoction thrice a day.

In **shooting pain in abdomen**—Take a paste of pieces of cinnamon bark with saunph seeds to avoid indigestion and relieve abdominal pain.

In **pyorrhoea**—To arrest foul odour emitting from the mouth, chew a piece of cinnamon bark thrice a day or hold a concentrated decoction of cinnamon in the mouth for 5 minutes after every meal.

Modern Studies

Anti fungal activity of cinnamon was clinically proven in patients of oral candidiasis in a study in New York.

Cinnamon is an important ingredient of a toothpaste found clinically effective in fighting dental disorders in a study at Udaipur.

In sex—To make sexual rejuvenation, take 3gm cinnamon with warm milk daily at night before sleep. It will increase the sperm count and also promote sexual stimulation.

24. Clove (Laung)

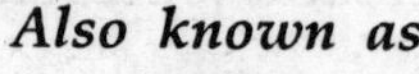

Also known as

Latin	:	Syzygium aromaticum
English	:	Clove
Sanskrit	:	Lavangam
Hindi	:	Laung
Marathi	:	Lavanga
Tamil	:	Kirampu
Telugu	:	Lavangamu
Malayalam	:	Karampu
Kannada	:	Lavanga

How it looks—It is a conical evergreen tree with a single main stem and sharp fragrant leaves. The flower buds are greenish to pink clustered at the ends of the branches and are highly aromatic. The fruits are fleshy and seeds are oval.

What we use—Dried flower buds.

What it does—It is aromatic, refrigerant, ophthalmic, digestive, carminative, stomachic, stimulant, anti-spasmodic, antibacterial, aphrodisiac, expectorant and anthelmintic.

How we use it—

In **vomiting**—Fry a couple of cloves, powder them and add a little honey to it for licking down slowly to stop vomiting.

In **stye**—In this eye infection, paste cloves and apply on the spot to reduce inflammation.

In **tooth cavity**—Drop a little clove juice into the dental cavity to numb the nerve endings and bring down pain. You could even chew the cloves as such for the same effect.

In **headaches**—Clove oil is a celebrated remedy for both headaches and toothaches. Even pasted cloves can be applied to the head as a counter irritant to relieve headaches.

In **coughs**—Even longstanding coughs can be rooted out by constantly chewing cloves. Some clove oil in a glass of hot milk will also serve the purpose.

To **subside thirst**—Especially in intestinal disorders when there is constant thirst, the peel of cloves should be pasted and taken with hot water.

Cloves contain a chemical called 'eugenol' that inhibits the growth of the bacteria. It is a natural antibiotic.

Modern Studies

Eugenol, an active principle of clove was found to inhibit gastric acid secretion in higher concentrations and facilitated digestion in lower concentrations.

Clove is an important ingredient of an ayurvedic tooth paste found clinically effective in combating dental disorders.

In **vomiting**—To curb vomiting in pregnant woman, boil 3gm cloves in 'kg water till water becomes half. Sip it slowly to check vomiting.

Modern Studies

Eugenol, an active principle of clove was found to inhibit gastric acid secretion in higher concentrations and facilitated digestion in lower concentrations.

Clove is an important ingredient of an ayurvedic tooth paste found clinically effective in combating dental disorders.

25. Coconut (Nariyal)

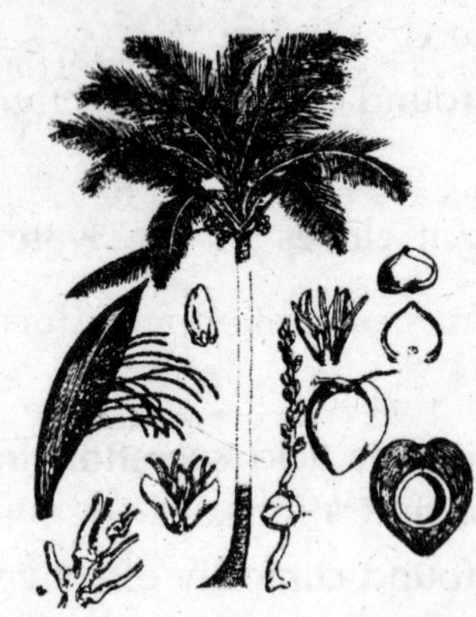

Also known as

Latin	**:**	**Cocos nucifera**
English	**:**	**Coconut**
Sanskrit	**:**	**Narikelah**
Hindi	**:**	**Nariyal**
Marathi	**:**	**Marala**
Tamil	**:**	**Tenkay**
Telugu	**:**	**Kobbarikaya**
Malayalam	**:**	**Nalikeram**
Kannada	**:**	**Tengu**

How it looks—It is a straight, graceful unbranched palm with a ringed stem bearing a crown of large leaves. The flowers are yellow or orange and contained in a longitudinally splitting sheath. The fruits are ovoid and green with a hard endocarp and oily white flesh with sweet milky or watery fluid in the large central cavity.

What we use—Roots, inflorescence, seeds (shell, kernel water and oil)

What it does—*Roots*—astringent, diuretic, anthelmintic.

Flower juice—sweet, refrigerant, aphrodisiac, intoxicating, diuretic and toxic.

Shell—cooling diuretic, deodorant

Kernel—sweet, cooling, oleaginous, appetiser, aphrodisiac, laxative and tonic.

Water—Sweet ,cooling, digestive, aphrodisiac, diuretic, anthelmintic and tonic.

Oil—Sweet, disinfectant, insecticidal, digestive, aphrodisiac, appetiser, hair tonic.

How we use it—

In **diarrhoea**—Coconut water is the ideal diet to replenish lost fluids.

In **urinary stones(gravel like)**—The flowers of coconut should be dried and powdered and taken along with yogurt.

In **headaches**—Tender coconut water relieves headache caused by overexposure to the sun.

In **worm infestations**—A decoction of the roots of coconut is taken with a pinch of asafoetida to rid oneself of intestinal worms.

In **wounds**—Old coconut oil is a quick healer of wounds.

In **vomiting**—Adding sugar ,honey and long pepper powder to tender coconut water makes a good preventive for vomiting.

Coconut milk—The milk of coconut makes an excellent body coolant on external application.

In **mouth ulcers**—The milk extracted from grated coconut makes a soothing and healing gargle for oral ulcers.

In **urticaria**—In generalised itching, coconut milk or even yogurt is applied to reduce inflammation.

In **scars**—Pasting the barks of banyan and peepal trees in coconut milk and applying over wounds helps skin heal smoothly owing to their, astringent and nourishing properties.

In **eczema**—Dried, shriveled garlic cloves are heated over low fire in coconut oil until the oil imbibes the black colour of the cloves. The cloves are then squeezed into the oil and the oil filtered. This makes an effective application over weeping eczematous lesions.

For **good hair growth**—Bathing the hair in coconut milk is an excellent practice to nourish hairs from roots to ends. This explains the well-nourished hair of people in Kerala, where this is a common practice.

Coconut oil has survived competition through decades and still remains the favourite base for many a commercial hair oil.

Post delivery—Dry coconut shavings, poppy seeds, dry ginger pieces, cucumber and pumpkin seeds are made into small sweet balls with jaggery. The newly delivered woman is given 1-2 of these balls daily.

Modern Studies

1. Tender coconut water was shown to be ideal even for intravenous administration in cases of dehydration and malnutrition.
2. Crude aqueous extract of the coir was found to show anti-bacterial effect against gram positive cocci (bacteria).

26. Coriander (Dhaniya)

Also known as

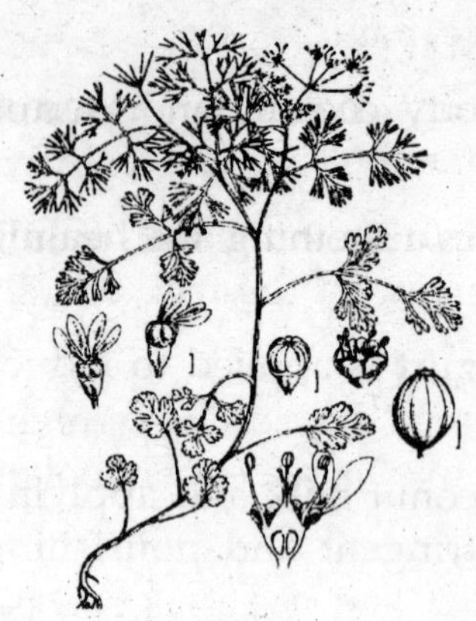

Latin	:	**Coriandrum sativum**
English	:	**Coriander**
Sanskrit	:	**Dhanyakam**
Hindi	:	**Dhaniya**
Marathi	:	**Dhane**
Tamil	:	**Kottamalli**
Telugu	:	**Dhaniyalu**
Malayalam	:	**Kottampala**
Kannada	:	**Kottambri**

The Sanskrit word "Dhanyaka" means "that which evokes praise while being eaten"

How it looks—It is an aromatic, much branched herb with small, white or pinkish purple flowers and yellowish brown, ribbed, 2- seeded fruits.

What we use—Fruits and leaves

What it does—*Leaves*—aromatic, analgesic, anti-inflammatory
Fruits—aromatic, digestive, carminative,styptic, anti-inflammatory, anthelmintic

How we use it—

In **excessive thirst**—Pasted coriander seeds are soaked in some water for a couple of hours and this water is taken with a little sugar and honey to quench long-standing thirst.

In **burning sensation**—Water prepared with coriander the same way as above is taken only with sugar in case of burning sensation either on the body or in passing urine.

In **jaundice**—Add 2 tsp of coriander seeds to a litre of water and add 2 tsp white cumin seeds to it. Leave this mixture overnight. On the next day , take a glass of this infusion twice or thrice a day after sweetening it with some palm candy. Repeat this for a couple of weeks until urine colour returns to normal.

In **fever**—Take "coriander tea" prepared with coriander decoction, very little milk and sugar. This causes sweating and brings down temperature.

In **gout**—Powder equal quantities of coriander and cumin seeds and add a sufficient amount of jaggery to it to make a confectionery. Make small balls of this and eat one thrice a day to get relief from the pain in gout.

In **indigestion and colicky pain**—Make a decoction of coriander seeds and dry ginger and consume thrice a day to stimulate digestion and relieve pain.

In **cough and breathing difficulty**—Mix a tsp of fine powder of coriander and saunph in a glass of rice wash to relieve cough and difficulty in breathing especially in children.

In **pregnancy**—Giving coriander decoction to the pregnant woman from the fifth month onwards promotes flow of urine and prevents oedema or swelling of the feet, usually noticed from that month of pregnancy onwards.

As a **coolant**—During summer, soak aniseeds, coriander seeds and poppy seeds overnight. In the morning, grind the seeds in the same water and filter it to obtain a super coolant drink for the body.

In **conjunctivitis**—Make a decoction of coriander seeds, cool it and use it as a wash for infected eyes to bring down pain and inflammation. Do this twice a day for a noticeable difference.

In high BP—To lower high blood pressure take coriander seeds, root of sarpgandha (*Rauwolfia serpentina*) and sugar candy in equal amount. Mix them and make powder. Take two teaspoonfuls with cold water twice a day.

27. Cumin (Jeera)

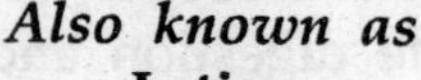

Also known as

Latin	**: Cuminum cyminum**
English	**: Cumin**
Sanskrit	**: Jiraka**
Hindi	**: Jeera**
Marathi	**: Jira**
Tamil	**: Jirakam**
Telugu	**: Jilakarra**
Malayalam	**: Jirakam**
Kannada	**: Jirige**

Jiraka means "fast acting" in Sanskrit.

How it looks—It is a small, slender annual herb with bluish green leaves, small white/ rose–coloured flowers and greyish fruits.

What we use—Fruits (though we call them cumin seeds they are actually the fruits of the plant)

What it does—It is cooling, anaphrodisiac, astringent, digestive, carminative, anthelmintic, anti-inflammatory, diuretic, galactogogue , and uterine and nervine tonic.

How we use it—

In **loss of appetite and flatulence**—Cumin powder and jaggery are rolled into small balls and consumed from time to time. Or you could make a decoction of the seeds to drink.

To increase breastmilk secretion—Take white cumin seeds fried in ghee with sugar for some days after delivery in doses of 1 tsp thrice daily with milk.

In **morning sickness**—For pregnant women, mix a tsp of cumin seed powder in some lime juice to drive nausea away.

In **white discharge**—Fry and powder cumin seeds and take a tsp twice a day with honey.

In **jaundice**—Leave a mixture of white cumin seeds in a vessel filled with water overnight. Sweeten this infusion with palm candy in the morning and drink it to increase urine output and to reduce fever.

In **colds and fevers**—Water boiled in cumin and ginger is used as a beverage to clear the infection.

In **boils**—A fine powder of cumin, mixed in coconut milk is applied over boils, especially in summer to effect a quick cure.

In **delayed periods**—A decoction of cumin and gingelly seeds, sweetened with palm candy, helps set off menstruation and promotes blood flow.

In **urinary calculi**—Take a tsp of cumin powder with sugar twice a day.

As a cosmetic—Wash the face with cumin-boiled water and then apply a paste of black and white cumin seeds in milk cream as a pack to clear and promote complexion.

Modern Study

Cumin was established as inhibiting platelet aggression in experimental studies..

28. Cutch tree (Khair)

Also known as

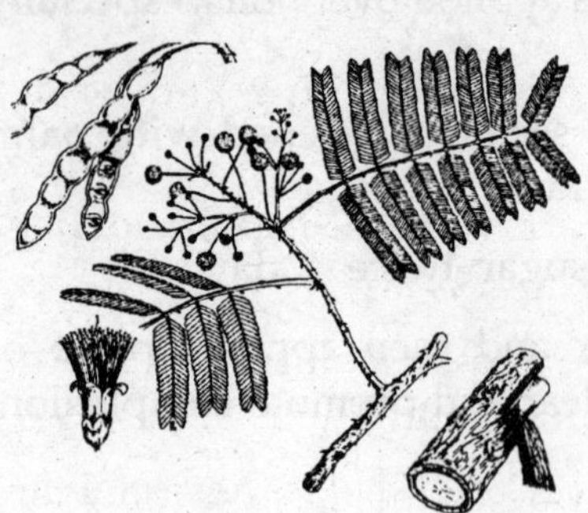

Latin	:	Acacia catechu
English	:	Cutch tree
Sanskrit	:	Khadirah
Hindi	:	Khair
Marathi	:	Khair
Tamil	:	Karunkali
Telugu	:	Podalimanu
Malayalam	:	Karinnali
Kannada	:	Kalu

"Which strengthens ṭeeth" is the meaning of the Sanskrit word "Khadirah".

How it looks—It is a moderate sized woody tree with dark greyish or brownish rough bark and hooked short spines. The leaves are bipinnately compound with a large gland near the middle of the main rachis. The flowers are pale yellow and the fruits are flat, brown, shiny pods enclosing 3-10 seeds each.

"Cutch" or "Kath" is the gummy extract of the wood which is available in a dark brown and brittle form. It is shiny on breaking and forms crystal-like pieces.

What we use—Bark, heartwood, kath

What it does—*Heartwood*—anthelmintic, cooling , antiseptic, antidysenteric, antipyretic, haemostatic, haematinic, anti-inflammatory.

Kath—thermogenic, digestive, appetiser, aphrodisiac, anthelmintic, depurative and tonic.

How we use it—

In **blood in sputum**—Gargle with a decoction of the bark and drink an ounce of it twice a day to stop blood appearing in sputum.

Tooth care—Boiling the powder of the heartwood in sesame oil and using it for gargling keeps all gum, tooth and other oral diseases at bay.

In **dry cough**—Mix a tsp of the powder of the heartwood with a cup of curd and swallow this preparation to soothe the throat. Khadir is excellent for all throat and voice disturbances. Hold the heartwood powder with some oil in the mouth for 5 minutes everyday.

In all **skin diseases**—It is a celebrated herbal drug for the cure of all skin diseases ranging from psoriasis and leprosy to eczema and common skin rashes. For best results, make a decoction of khadir heartwood and amla powder and drink an ounce twice a day.

Water boiled with khadir powder should be used for drinkin, bathing and washing the patches.

In **tooth disorders**—Gargle with the decoction of khadir everyday to keep free of dental caries, gum infections and tooth disorders.

In **diabetes**—Take an ounce of the decoction of Khadira and arecanut every morning to regulate urination and keep blood sugar levels under control.

In **toxic states**—In suspicion of any poisoning, drink water with the root powder of khadir and powdered neem seeds immediately.

Modern Study

Hepato protective activity of ethyl acetate extract of acacia catechu was demonstrated in experimental studies on albino rats in Trivandrum.

29. Dates/Khajur

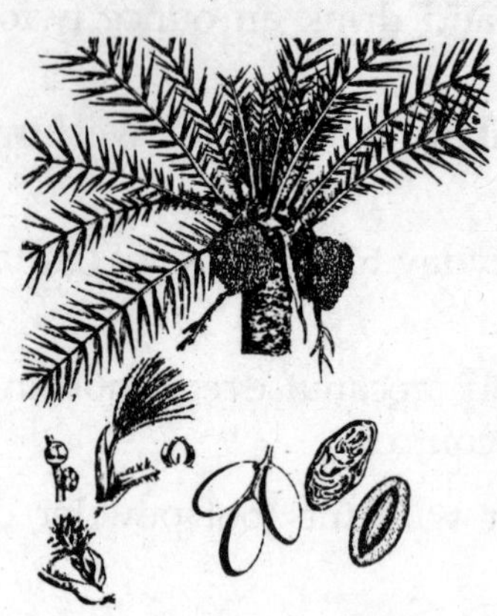

Also known as

Latin	:	Phoenix dactylifera
English	:	Dates
Sanskrit	:	Kharjurah
Hindi	:	Khajur
Marathi	:	Khajura
Tamil	:	Periccankay
Telugu	:	Karjurakaya
Malayalam	:	Ittappana
Kannada	:	Kajjuri

How it looks—It is a tall palm growing up to 36 m in length with its trunk covered by the bases of petioles. The leaves are pinnate as in all palms but the lower ones are modified into spines and the flowers are in spadices. The fruits are oval, reddish or yellowish brown berries with fleshy sweet pulp and hard single furrowed seeds.

What we use—Leaves, flowers, fruits, seeds

What it does—*Leaves* — aphrodisiac, hepato protective
Flowers — purgative, expectorant, hepatic, febrifuge
Fruits — cooling, aphrodisiac, tonic, diuretic, anti-anaemic

How we use it—

In **cough, and respiratory disorders**—Make a paste of dates, raisins, pepper, saunph seeds, honey and ghee and lick a tsp of this preparation twice a day to expectorate phlegm and calm respiratory spasms.

In **dryness of mouth**—At the end of long duration of an illness, the mouth becomes dry, sore making swallowing and talking difficult. In such cases, make a paste of dates and raisins and coat the mouth with it. Hold the same paste in the mouth for a few minutes and eat it with honey and ghee.

In **hiccups**—Powder the seeds of dates, mix it with pepper powder and lick it with honey to arrest hiccups.

In **excessive bleeding**—Dates are cooling and bestow blood and are therefore ideal in bleeding conditions. Paste the fruit with honey and eat twice a day.

In **constipation**—Soak dates in hot milk for a few hours and then take the preparation at bed time to free bowel movements. Dates soaked in water make excellent diuretics.

As a **nervine tonic**—Dates and raisins pasted with honey are excellent in nervous disorders and can be taken as a general rejuvenator.

In **forgetfulness**—Dates are also reported to be used in cases of memory disturbance.

30. Deodar/Devdar

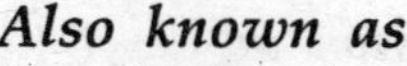

Also known as

Latin	:	Cedrus deodara
English	:	Deodar
Sanskrit	:	Devadaru
Hindi	:	Devdar
Marathi	:	Deodara
Tamil	:	Tevataram
Telugu	:	Devadari
Malayalam	:	Devataram
Kannada	:	Devadari

How it looks—It is a tall graceful coniferous tree with black, furrowed bark found in the Himalayas.The cones are found at the end of branches, with pale brown seeds. The heartwood of deodar is yellowish brown turning brown on exposure. It is oily, fragrant and strong.

What we use—Leaves, heartwood, oil

What it does—*Leaves*—anti-inflammatory, antitubercular,

Heartwood—anthelmentic, digestive, carminative, cardiotonic anti-inflammatory, diuretic, expectorant, antiseptic.

Oil—antiseptic, depurative, diuretic.

How we use it—

In **hiccough and breathlessness**—Make a decoction with pieces of deodar wood and drink twice a day to clear airways and soothe the diaphragm which causes hiccough.

In **wounds, leprosy, syphilis**—Being antiseptic and antiphlogistic, it is used externally as a hot paste with water. It is also a well-known blood purifier and deodar oil can be taken internally in the above cases.

In **filariasis**—Make a paste of deodar with some mustard oil and apply on the affected part to fight obstruction to the vessels and reduce swelling. Deodar is especially recommended in glandular diseases.

As a **diuretic**—Drink the decoction of deodar wood twice a day to promote urination and clear urinary obstruction. This decoction is also used with great benefits in fever.

Modern Study

The oil of deodar was found to possess significant anti-inflammatory activity in experimental studies.

31. Dhub Grass (Durba)

Also known as

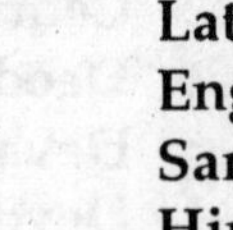

Latin	:	**Cynodon dactylon**
English	:	**Dhub Grass, Conch Grass**
Sanskrit	:	**Durva**
Hindi	:	**Durba**
Marathi	:	**Durva**
Tamil	:	**Arukampallu**
Telugu	:	**Garika**
Malayalam	:	**Karuka**
Kannada	:	**Garika hallu**

How it looks—It is a prostate extensively creeping perennial grass highly branched and rooting at every node. The leaves are narrow and linear and the inflorescence is in terminal spikes and green or purplish in colour. The fruit grains are oblong and compressed at the sides.

What we use—Whole plant

What it does—It is haemostatic, cooling, depurative, constipating ,diuretic and tonic.

How we use it—

In **stings and bites**—Boil a handful of the grass in about a litre of water and reduce to half. Drink this decoction to flush out toxins from the system.

In **eczema**—You can prepare a medicated oil by boiling in coconut oil a handful of dhub grass, a few sticks of liquorice and some harad powder. This oil must be applied daily before bath.

For **hair growth**—Paste dhub grass, liquorice and harad and boil this in coconut oil until the paste chars. Filter it and use regularly to nourish hair and stimulate growth.

In **burns**—Prepare a medicated oil by boiling dhub grass in coconut oil and adding myrrh or Guggulu prices to it. The filtered oil is highly coolant and injures rapid healing of burnt skin.

In **infertility**—Taking half a cup of the juice of dhub grass everyday is said to correct reproductive disorders and facilitate conception. This is also used as a preventive against abortions.

In **bleeding disorders**—The juice expressed from the fresh dhub plant is highly coolant and haemostatic and therefore helps arrest bleeding immediately.

In **urinary disorders**—Being highly diuretic, the diluted and sweetened juice of dhub grass clears urinary obstruction of any kind and establishes free flow of urine.

As a **brain tonic**—Dhub grass is known for its intellect promoting property and is a component of many a brain tonic preparation. Here too, the fresh juice is taken in doses of an ounce everyday.

32. Drumstick (Sahijan)

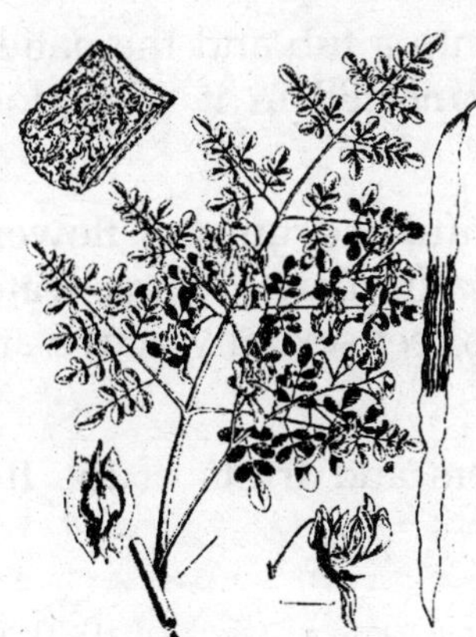

Also known as

Latin	**:**	**Moringa oleifera**
English	**:**	**Drumstick**
Sanskrit	**:**	**Sigruh, Sobhanjanah**
Hindi	**:**	**Sahijan**
Marathi	**:**	**Sheraga**
Tamil	**:**	**Murunkai**
Telugu	**:**	**Munaga**
Malayalam	**:**	**Muringa**
Kannada	**:**	**Nuggi, Murunga**

How it looks—It is a middle sized tree with grey bark and brittle branches. It has rounded leaves, white flowers and typical long fruit pods, with 3-sided seeds.

What we use—Roots, bark, leaves, seeds

What it does—*Roots*—digestive, carminative, constipating, expectorant

Bark—thermogenic, abortifacient, antifungal, cardiac stimulant

Leaves—anti-inflammatory, anthelmintic

Seeds—anti-inflammatory, purgative

How we use it—

In **stomach ulcers**—The leaves are ground into a paste mixed in curd and taken daily.

In **sore throat**—Apply a fine paste of drumstick leaves with a pinch of lime at the base of the throat at bedtime. Combine this therapy with a salt water gargle.

In **mouth ulcers**—Take drumstick leaves liberally to cure mouth ulcers.

In **hiccough and breathing disorders**—Make a decoction of the leaves and drink twice a day to obtain relief.

In **running nose**—Inhale the vapours of the roots boiled in water to clear the nasal passages and bring out obstructing mucous.

In **worm infestations**—The decoction of the bark along with honey acts as a good anthelmintic.

In **unripe abscess**—All the parts of the drumstick tree are useful in an abscess in which pus does not form. Drinking the bark decoction, eating the fruit, and making a topical application of the leaves are all highly beneficial.

In **itching**—Apply a paste of the roots to relieve itching.

In **urinary stones**—Make a decoction of the peel of the roots and drink it thrice daily, to break down small urinary stones naturally.

In **non-bleeding piles**—The decoction of the bark is poured into a tub and the patient asked to sit in it in such a way that the pile masses are immersed in it. This done regularly prevents bleeding and shrinks the pile masses.

To **increase sexual vigour**—Make a preparation of a tablespoonful of drumstick flowers, one egg white, 2 dates, 4 grated almonds and a pinch of saffron with some water. Take this preparation thrice a week for a couple of months to feel sexually active and vigorous.

To **increase resistance**—Make a curry with the leaves flowers and fruits of the tree to prevent frequent infections.

Modern Studies

1. Aqueous and alcoholic extracts of the root and flower of Moringa oleifera were found to have antihepatotoxic (liver protective) activity on paracetamol- treated rats in a study in Trichy, Tamil Nadu.
2. In another study in Vadodara, the stem bark was shown to possess oedema – suppressant activity.
3. In yet another study on mice in the Philippines, the seed extracts of Moringa oliefera were shown to possess anti-inflammatory and antitumour activities.

33. Euphorbiaceae (Jamgliamli)

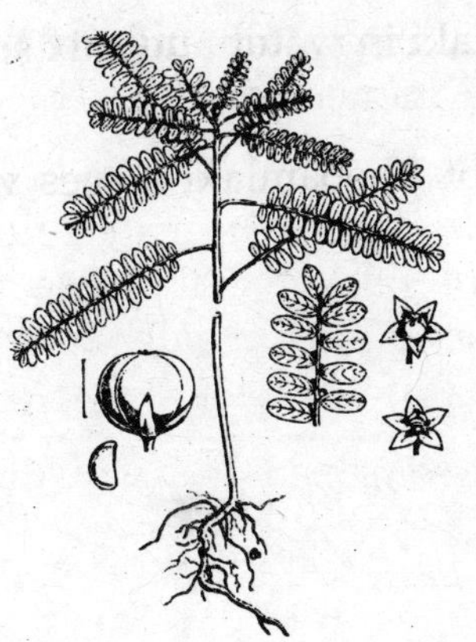

Also known as

Latin	:	Phyllanthus neruri
English	:	Euphorbiaceae
Sanskrit	:	Tamalaki, Bhumyamlaki
Hindi	:	Jamgliamli
Marathi	:	Bhuianwla
Tamil	:	Kilanelli
Telugu	:	Nelausiriki
Malayalam	:	Kilarnelli
Kannada	:	Kirunelli

How it looks—It is a branching annual glabrous herb with slender spreading branchlets. The leaves are numerous with a rounded base. The flowers are yellowish, greenish or whitish in colour. Fruits are rounded smooth capsules with trigonous seeds.

What we use—Whole plant

What it does—It is sweet, diuretic, febrifuge, astringent and antiseptic.

How we use it—

In **jaundice**—In all liver disorders, take a concentrated decoction of the leaves of Bhoomlaki every morning for six days. It is highly hepatoprotective.

Once jaundice is cured, fry the berries of makoi (manthakkali in Tamil & Malayalam) in ghee and mix this with rice and eat at the beginning of every meal to improve digestion and general resistance.

In **fevers**—An infusion of the leaves every morning brings down temperature especially in intermittent fevers, being cooling, and febrifuge.

In **diarrhoea and dysentery**—Mix the paste of the leaves with some fenugreek seeds and curds and swallow this mixture to arrest loose motions immediately.

In **scabies**—Being antiseptic, an application of pasted Bhooamlaki leaves on infected skin and on wounds effects quick healing.

In **urinary infections**—In any disorders of the urinary system, Bhooamlaki is helpful in the form of a cooled decoction, twice a day, owing to its coolant and diuretic properties.

In **thirst and burning sensation**—Apply a cool paste of the leaves on hands and feet to soothe burning sensation and drink an infusion of the leaves to mitigate long-standing thirst. In burning sensation in the eyes or any other eye disorder a few drops of the juice of the leaves are instilled in the eyes. Again, its antiseptic property comes into play to effect a quick cure.

In **white discharge and menstrual disorders**—Grind the seeds of Bhooamlaki in rice wash and drink every day for a few weeks to get rid of the above afflictions.

In **hiccough and breathlessness**—Paste the roots of Bhooamlaki in water and mix some saumph seeds in it before drinking.

In **diabetes**—When blood sugar has shot up, take a fistful of Bhooamlaki leaves with a tsp of black pepper powder everyday for a week.

34. Fennel (Saunph)

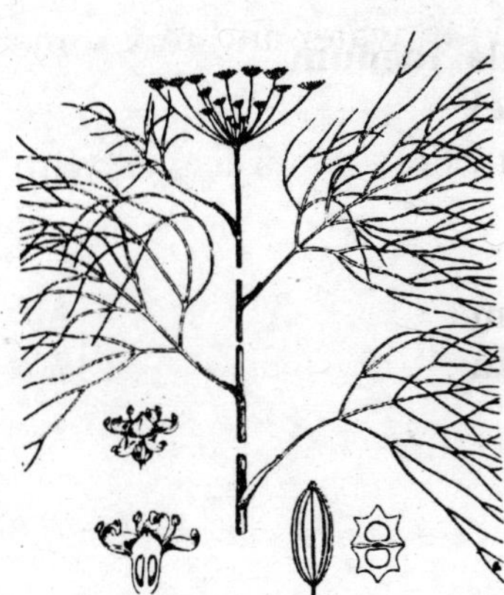

Also known as

Latin	:	**Foeniculum vulgare**
English	:	**Fennel**
Sanskrit	:	**Misreya**
Hindi	:	**Saunph**
Marathi	:	**Sop**
Tamil	:	**Sompu**
Telugu	:	**Peddajeelakarra**
Malayalam	:	**Perumjirakam**
Kannada	:	**Badhesuppu**

How it looks—It is a stiff, aromatic herb, with narrow leaves, and small, fragrant yellow flowers. The fruits are oval/cylindrical and yellowish brown in colour.

What we use—Fruits

What it does—*Fruits*—refrigerant expectorant, anthelmintic, carminative, digestive, cardiac stimulant, galactogogue, diuretic

How we use it—

To **increase breastmilk secretion**—Pound a few saunph seeds into a glass of milk and give everyday to a lactating mother for promotion of milk secretion.

In **vomiting**—Crush a few ginger pieces and some saunph seeds and add to half a glass of boiling water and allow to cool. Drink this water from time to time to suppress nausea and vomiting.

As a **digestive**—Commonly used as a mouth freshener after meals, saunph is basically a digestive. Chewing a few seeds after a meal clears the food passages ,apart from aiding digestion.

Modern Study

Anethole, an extract of fennel was found to reduce fructose concentrations and thereby prostate gland weight in experimental studies.

35. Fenugreek (Methi)

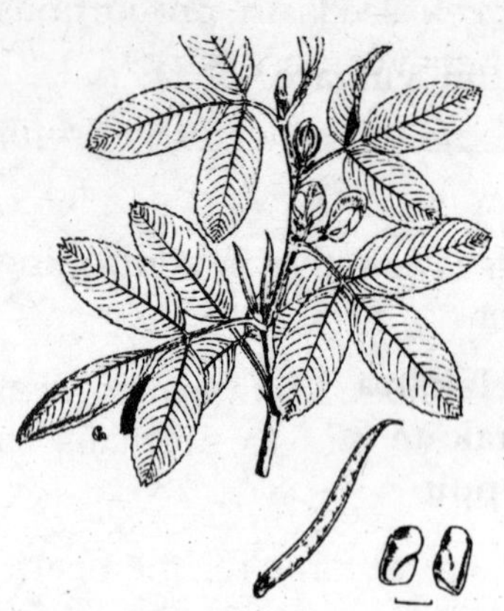

Also known as

Latin	**:**	**Trigonella foenum**
English	**:**	**Fenugreek**
Sanskrit	**:**	**Methika**
Hindi	**:**	**Methi**
Marathi	**:**	**Methi**
Tamil	**:**	**Ventayam**
Telugu	**:**	**Menthulu**
Malayalam	**:**	**Uluva**
Kannada	**:**	**Mentya**

How it looks—It is an aromatic, erect annual herb with pinnate, leaves and toothed leaflets. The flowers are white or yellowish white and the fruits are pods with many seeds.

What we use—Leaves, seeds

What it does—*Leaves*—refrigerant, aperient

Seeds—mucilaginous, aromatic, carminative, tonic, galactogogue, astringent, anaphrodisiac.

How we use it—

In **griping abdominal pain**—A tsp of powdered fenugreek seeds mixed in buttermilk helps digestion and relieves pain

In **flatulence**—Crush a few fenugreek seeds with a pinch of rock salt for quick relief from flatulence.

In **piles & oral ulcers**—Including fenugreek leaves in plenty in the diet of a piles patient is useful.

In **eruptive fevers**—Give plenty of fenugreek water during the early stages of small pox, chicken pox or measles. (A tsp of the seeds is soaked in a pint of water overnight to prepare fenugreek water). The alkaloid trigonelline in fenugreek is antiseptic and carminative.

In **dandruff**—2 tsp of fenugreek seeds are soaked overnight in water and the softened seeds are ground and left on the scalp for ½ hour to get rid of dandruff.

In **eczema**—After washing the lesions with a solution of tea and rock salt, the part is dried and covered with a dilute paste of fenugreek and red sandal.

To **clean skin**—A mixture of green gram, bengal gram and fenugreek seeds makes a good substitute for soap.

As a **shampoo**—Similarly, shikakai green gram and fenugreek seeds in proportions of 2:1:1/2 are powdered together and used with water whenever necessary.

In **joint stiffness**—Drinking a tsp of fenugreek powder in some warm water is useful in preventing tightness of the joints.

In **white vaginal discharge**—Methi powder mixed with curds is effective in controlling infection. The same recipe is a tested remedy for diarrhoea.

After **delivery**—Fry fenugreek seeds in ghee and finely powder them. Mix this in wheat flour and sugar and make a halwa- like preparation. This is proved to normalise a woman's system after delivery. Dosa-1 table spoon every day.

In **heart problems**—Fenugreek seeds in water everyday is a natural tonic for the heart..

As a **body coolant and tonic**—Rice/starch water with a tsp of fenugreek powder is an excellent body coolant

Modern Studies

Recently animal studies have shown the effectiveness of fenugreek in reducing blood pressure.

As a diet in pregnancy, diabetes and anaemia, it has proved to be nourishing and vitalising.

36. Fig (Anjeer)

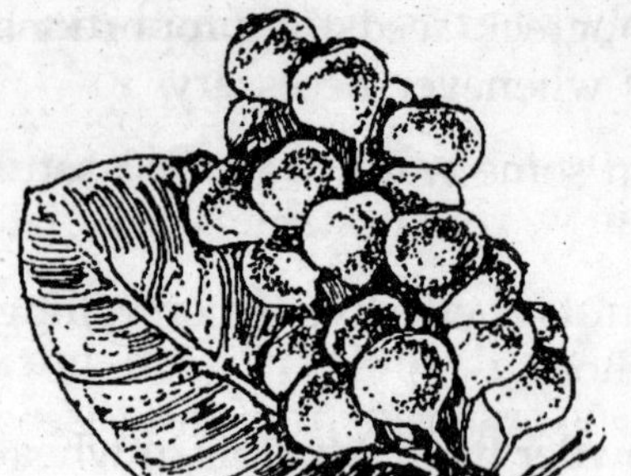

Also known as

Latin	:	**Ficus carica**
English	:	**Fig**
Sanskrit	:	**Anjeera**
Hindi	:	**Anjeer**
Marathi	:	**Anjeer**
Tamil	:	**—**
Telugu	:	**—**
Malayalam	:	**—**
Kannada	:	**Anjeera**

Fig is a tree brought to India during the Moghul rule and has stayed over since. The leaves are highly useful as feed for cattle.

How it looks—It is a medium sized tree with leaves rough on the upper surface and softer on the under surfaces. The fruits arise from the corners of the leaves and turn red in colour when ripe. They are many seeded. The latex of the tree is used medicinally.

What we use—*Fruit latex*

What it does—It is highly nutritive, diuretic, expectorant, laxative Figs are high sources of calcium, iron and copper. Zinc is also moderately present. Vit. A and C are present in all forms of fig fruit while Vit. A is lost by 30% in dry ones.

Vit B complex and vit D are also present.

How we use it—

In **delayed periods**—Boil the roots of the fig and take the decoction, filtered for a few weeks to set the cycle normal.

In **urinary stones and dysuria**—Boil figs in water to get a decoction. Take an ounce or two of this decoction twice a day to set right urinary disorders and to melt small stones.

In **burn ulcers**—Boil the bark of fig in water along with neem, mango and peepal barks. This decoction is very useful to wash and soothe ulcers caused by burns.

To **build resistance**—Take a dry fig fruit or two everyday to build body resistance and for your natural daily requirement of vitamins.

In **anaemia**—Due to the iron-rich content of fig, it is ideal to include it in one's diet in anaemia.

In **hyperacidity**—The burnt ash of the fig fruit is highly basic in nature and can be consumed a tsp before meals to counter hyperacidity.

In **worm infestation**—The enzyme ficin present in the fig latex is responsible for its anthelmintic activity and can be given with great benefit in worm infestations especially ascaris and tricharus types.

In **leucoderma**—Fig is used in white spots on skin as it contains a chemical *"furocoumarin"* which is responsible for this action. A person suffering from this disease is advised to take fig in any form for 2/3 months.

In **amoebiasis**—Sherbat or Ark anjir available in the market is use' to cure amoebiasis.

37. Garlic (Lahsun)

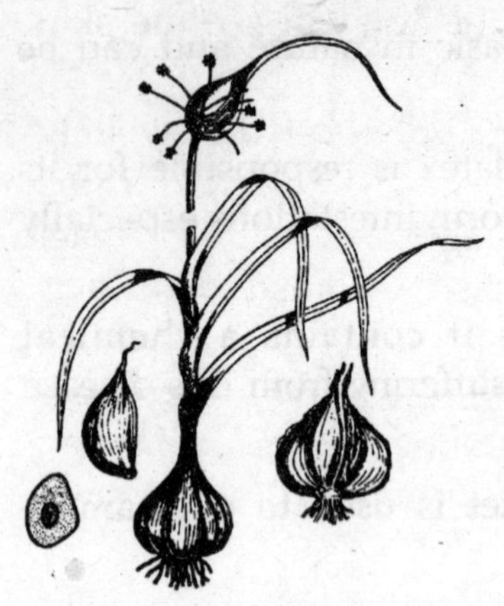

Also known as

Latin	:	**Allium cepa**
English	:	**Garlic**
Sanskrit	:	**Lasunah, Rasonah**
Hindi	:	**Lahsun**
Marathi	:	**Lasuna**
Tamil	:	**Vellaipuntu**
Telugu	:	**Velluli, Tellagadda**
Malayalam	:	**Velluli**
Kannada	:	**Bellili**

> **The very word "lashuna" in sanskrit means "that which devours diseases of the heart"**

How it looks—It is a perennial herb with simple long, flat leaves, small white flowers and white bulb-like rhizomes.

What we use—*Bulbs.*

What it does—It is stimulant, anticholesterol, antibacterial, aphrodisiac, analgesic, anthelmintic, diuretic, emmenagogue and antifungal.

How we use it—

In seasonal fevers—Mix a few cloves of garlic with some til oil or ghee and take it before a warm nutritious meal to bring down fever of any type.

In epileptic fits—The usage of the same preparation of garlic cloves with oil should be taken daily in cases of epilepsy.

In infected wounds—Make a fine paste of garlic cloves and apply on wounds to rid them of worms. Roll the paste into a ball and leave it on the wound.

In earaches—Instill a few drops of the juice of garlic cloves in the aching ear, or crush a few cloves of garlic in some til oil and instill the same into the ear.

In joint pains, high cholesterol and heart disease—Boil a few crushed cloves in a glass of milk and four glasses of water and reduce it to a glass. Take this preparation every day for about 40 days and feel the difference.

In asthma and respiratory allergies—Take some ginger tea with some garlic cloves in it, twice a day to reduce susceptibility to allergies and clear airways.

In **eczema**—Store garlic cloves which have been dried in shade for a long time. For weeping lesions, boil some of these in some coconut oil until the cloves turn black. Squeeze out these charred cloves into the oil and apply. You can see the skin turn healthy within a few weeks.

In sprains—Paste some garlic and turmeric in quicklime and apply over the swelling to reduce pain and inflammation.

In joint pain—Crush some garlic cloves in green gram soup and take daily for relief from pain and stiffness. In cold regions, garlic cloves crushed in mustard oil acts as a warming and stimulating application.

To increase breastmilk secretion—Garlic is usually included in considerable quantities in a newly delivered mother's diet for its lactogenic effect amongst other properties. However, if the child develops diarrhoea or any other complication, its use should be discontinued.

To revive consciousness : Squeezing a few drops of garlic juice into a fainted person's nostrils usually restores consciousness.

In abdominal distension—Garlic soup is the best recommended medicine to relieve a gas—distended abdomen. Crush a few garlic cloves in some Bengal gram water to make the soup. Cumin, pepper and coriander seeds may be added for potency.

Modern Studies

1. Raw garlic juice and the extract of garlic have shown anti-stress effects in experimental studies.
2. A 42-year old female patient suffering from candidiasis (fungal infection in vagina) was completely cured by daily administration of 4-5 garlic cloves for 4 months.
3. Raw garlic paste mixed in cow butter as an oral administration was clinically proven to be an effective remedy in Bell's palsy or facial palsy.
4. Daily intake of raw garlic prevents rise of blood cholesterol levels.
5. In a clinical study consisting of 114 human patients with clear cut hypertension and Atherosclerosis, it was observed that an overwhelming majority of patients responded favourably to the garlic therapy.
6. In experiments on animals and human workers exposed to chronic lead intoxication, garlic has been found to be an efficacious preventive as well as curative drug.
7. In cancer, it is found to be effective. Transplanted tumours of Jensen sarcoma in rats regressed, and in some cases, completely disappeared after the injection of 1-3 mg of 'Allicin', an active fraction of garlic was given directly into the tumour. However, all types of tumours do not respond equally well.
8. Decreases incidence of thrombus formation.
9. It is found to be anti-amoebic and its action is equivalent to that of Metronidezole.
10. Activates prostatic function and increases sexual ability.

38. Gingelly/Til

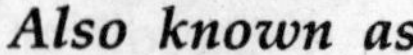

Also known as

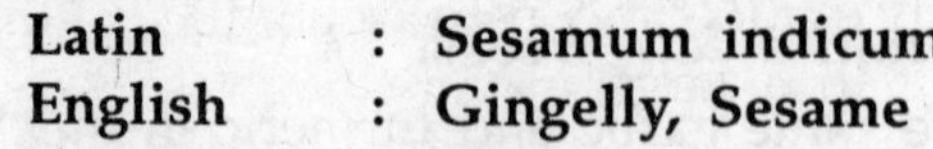

Latin	:	**Sesamum indicum**
English	:	**Gingelly, Sesame**
Sanskrit	:	**Tilah**
Hindi	:	**Til**
Marathi	:	**Tila**
Tamil	:	**Ellu, Eellu-cceti**
Telugu	:	**Nuvvulu**
Malayalam	:	**Ellu**
Kannada	:	**Ellu**

How it looks—It is an erect, annual plant with large thin leaves, white, pink or purplish flowers and quadrangular oval fruits

What we use—Roots, leaves, seeds, oil

What it does—*Roots & leaves*—emollient

Seeds—astringent, laxative, thermogenic, aphrodisiac, galactogogue, digestive, hair restorer, tonic,

Oil— astringent, anthelmintic, constipating, thermogenic

How we use it—

In **joint pains**—Leave a tsp of black gingelly seeds in a glass of water overnight, and drink it in a morning.

Alternately, a tsp of gingelly seeds with ½ a tsp of dry ginger powder should be taken with a glass of hot milk every morning.

To induce puberty—In underdeveloped adolescent girls, it is useful to give a decoction of til seeds everyday. (or) Gingelly seeds and jaggery are rolled into small "laddoos"and are taken one thrice a day to stimulate overall physical development and for increasing lactation **in breastfeeding women**.

In **dysmenorrhoea**—The same gingelly jaggery laddoos or any preparation with gingelly is useful to promote free flow of menstrual blood and ease pain and discomfort accompanying menstrual flow.

In **bedwetting**—Half a tsp of gingelly with a quarter tsp of ajowain should be given to the child at night along with mineral water. Even gingelly-jaggery laddoos can be given according to the age of the child.

In **high blood pressure**—Gingelly oil can substitute other cooking media such as ghee, groundnut oil, coconut oil, mustard oil or even refined oil, as til oil retains all its natural benefits besides having the least amount of saturated fat.

In **piles**—Especially in bleeding, using a poultice of the seeds pasted with butter relieves pain and bleeding to a large extent.

In **gout**—Steam boiling sesame seeds and pasting with milk makes an effective application on gouty joints.

In **diarrhoea**—Black sesame seeds are pasted with a dash of sugar and eaten along with goat milk.

In **colicky pain**—Rolling a ball made of sesame seed pasted over the abdomen soothes the shooting pain.

In **cracked heels/soles**—Applying gingelly oil on the affected area and fomenting the feet with hot water at night is highly beneficial.

For jet black hair—Black sesame seeds, amla and bhringraj powdered together and applied maintain the rich black texture of hair besides completely revitalizing it.

For **strong teeth**—Chewing a handful of sesame seeds and washing it down with cool water regularly will ensure a set of healthy teeth. Gargling with sesame oil everyday is just as effective.

Modern Study

The external application of sesame oil was found to exhibit anti-cancer activity in malignant melanoma in an experimental study.

39. Ginger (Adarakh)

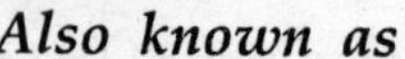

Also known as

Latin	**:**	**Zingiber officinarum**
English	**:**	**Ginger**
Sanskrit	**:**	**Ardrakam**
Hindi	**:**	**Adarak**
Marathi	**:**	**Ale**
Tamil	**:**	**Inci**
Telugu	**:**	**Allamu**
Malayalam	**:**	**Erukkilangu, inji**
Kannada	**:**	**Hasisunti**

How it looks—It is a slender, perennial, rhizomatous herb, with yellowish green flowers and long leaves. The rhizomes are white to yellowish brown in colour and irregularly branched.

What we use—Rhizomes (raw and dry states)

What it does—*Raw*—thermogenic, carminative, laxative, digestive

Dry—thermogenic, appetiser, laxative, stomachic, stimulant, aphrodisiac, expectorant, anthelmentic, carminative

How we use it—

To improve appetite and digestion—Mix Trikatu (rock salt, pepper and long pepper) in some ginger juice and gargle a few times to acquire a strong appetite and power of digestion.

In **indigestion**—The decoction of dry ginger and rock salt is very helpful in tackling undigested material

In **jaundice**—Take a tsp of powder of dry ginger with some jaggery twice a day for free passage of stools and as a liver tonic.

In **ascites**—Take equal quantities of ginger juice and milk every day after both your meals.

In **diarrhoea**—Boil dry ginger and khaskhas roots in a glass of water and take thrice a day to arrest loose motions.

In **cholera**—Add some dry ginger powder to decoction of the flesh of bael fruits and take this twice a day to arrest vomiting and diarrhoea.

In **piles**—Make small balls of dry ginger and jaggery and eat one twice a day to reduce the masses and allow free passage of stools.

In **colicky pain**—Equal parts of sonth, til seeds and jaggery should be pasted and drunk with milk twice a day.

In **colds / asthmatic attacks**—Ginger tea—Crushed ginger is added to water boiling for tea and tea is prepared with this water .Take this tea to decrease inflammation and relieve congestion and body ache.

In **asthma,** a few garlic cloves my be added to the above tea. Ginger may be mixed with mustard oil and applied externally on the chest to relieve congestion.

In **ear aches**—Warm a little ginger juice and instill a few drops in the ear to relieve pain and clear infected material.

In **arthritic joints**—A decoction of dry ginger and castor roots should be taken every morning for lubrication of joints and relief from pain.

In **blood in urine**—Boil 1 tsp of dry ginger in a glass of milk and drink twice a day to arrest the bleeding.

In **allergic rashes**—Crush some old jaggery in ginger juice and take twice a day to soothe the rashes.

In **hiccough**—Mix jaggery and ginger juice and instill a few drops in the nostrils to stop hiccups.

In **heart disease**—Take a hot decoction of dry ginger after the morning meal daily to keep heart disease in check.

In **toothaches**—Apply a paste of dry ginger on the outside of the cheek at the point of pain.

On **stings**—Dry ginger paste mixed in yogurt is an effective topical application to reduce the swelling.

In **scrotal swelling**—Apply a mixture of dry ginger and salt solution on hydroceles to reduce pain and swelling.

Modern Studies

Experimental studies proved that ginger juice and its extracts improved gastric emptying and thereby were effective against gastro-intestinal disturbances.

It was shown that ginger along with garlic significantly reduces blood glucose and serum lipids in experimental studies on rats.

40. Gooseberry (Amla)

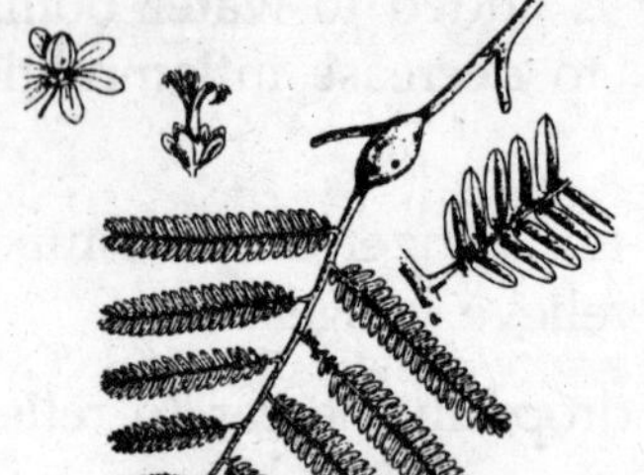

Also known as

Latin	:	**Emblica officinalis**
English	:	**Gooseberry**
Sanskrit	:	**Amalaki, Dhatri**
Hindi	:	**Amla**
Marathi	:	**Anwla**
Tamil	:	**Nelli**
Telugu	:	**Usirikaya**
Malayalam	:	**Nellimaram**
Kannada	:	**Nellaka**

The Sanskrit name "Amalaki" means "that which is full of rejuvenating properties".

How it looks—It is a small to medium sized woody tree, with light grey bark and many tiny closely set leaves. The flowers are greenish yellow and fruits are rounded, pale yellow and fleshy with 3-sided seeds.

What we use—Root bark, bark, leaves, fruits

What it does— *Root bark*—astringent

Fruits—sour, astringent, cooling, opthalmic, carminative, digestive, laxative, aphrodisiac, diuretic, antipyretic.

How we use it—

In **recurrent nasal infections**—Take a diet of rice mixed with amla powder, mustard powder and a pinch of rock salt regularly to prevent frequent attacks of cold and sinusitis.

In **hair care**—A most celebrated hair conditioner, a quarter kilo of amla fruits are boiled in a kilo of coconut oil and stored to make an effective preventive for balding and greying of hair.

In **oily hair**—Take half a cup of amla juice and half a cup of lime juice and dilute this to make an anti-grease hair wash.

To **arrest bleeding**—Drink the fresh juice of amla fruits diluted in water, or mix a tsp of amla powder in a glass of water and drink from time to time to check bleeding.

As a **coolant**—Gooseberries are boiled in coconut oil and massaged over the scalp during summer for its coolant activity.

You could also pickle gooseberries and include in your diet during summer. This practice is prevalent especially in South India.

In **white spots on the nails**—Gooseberry is an excellent source of Vit-C and so serves as an effective remedy in vitamin-deficient conditions.

In **anaemia**—Add amla juice and honey to sugarcane juice and drink everyday to ward off anaemia.

In **bleeding piles**—Take the watery part of yogurt and add some amla juice to it. Drink this mixture twice daily to arrest bleeding in piles.

In **white discharge**—Powder the dry seeds of amla and take a tsp of it with some honey and saunph seeds twice daily.

Alternatively, you could also take a ripe banana and mix a tsp of amla seed powder and eat everyday.

In **colic pain**—Mix a tsp of saunph powder in half a cup of amla juice and drink to relieve shooting abdominal pain.

In **hoarse voice and cough**—Add a tsp of amla powder to a glass of warm milk and drink thrice a day to clear an unpleasant throat. In dry cough, add some ghee to the above preparation before drinking.

In **dysentery**—Squeeze the juice out of a handful of amla leaves into a glass of milk. Add some honey and ghee to this milk and drink to stop loose motions accompanied by mucous and/or blood.

In **diabetes**—Probably the most celebrated effect of amla is its anti-diabetic property. Take ¼ cup of amla fruit juice or a tsp of amla powder with a tsp of turmeric powder everyday.

For **skin tone**—After brushing, hold the decoction of amla fruits in your mouth for 3-5 minutes and sprinkle the same into your eyes. This procedure done regularly, renders you free of dryness and discolourations of the skin and boils.

As a **health tonic**—As one of the richest sources of Vit-C, amla can be used generally to prevent infections and tone up the body.

An **effective recipe**—Powder dry gooseberry fruits with an equal number of dry dates and seedless raisins and some sugar candy crystals. Roll this preparation into small pills and take a pill every day as a general rejuvenator.

Modern Study

Gooseberry was shown to be an effective food supplement during the treatment of Insulin Dependent Diabetes Mellitus, at a study in Coimbatore.

41. Grapes (Angoor)

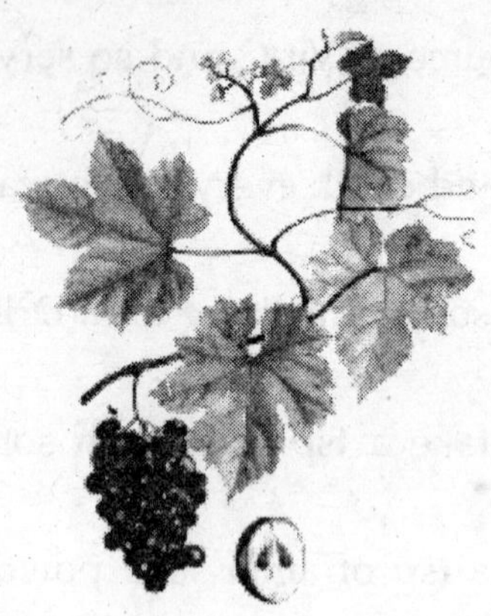

Also known as

Latin	:	**vitis vinifera**
English	:	**Common grape-vine,**
Sanskrit	:	**Draksha**
Hindi	:	**Dakh, Angoor**
Marathi	:	**Drakshe/Angoora**
Tamil	:	**Tiratchai**
Telugu	:	**Draksha**
Malayalam	:	**Muntiri**
Kannada	:	**Draksha**

Introduction—The grape is a very important sub-tropical fruit in the world with 80% of its cultivation contributing to wine making, 10% to raisins and only 10% sold as fresh fruit. Raisin grapes must have a sugar content of 24-28 percent, usually not found in India; which grows grapes with sugar levels of 13-22%.

How it looks—It is a slender turning climber, with 3-5 lobed leaves. Flowers are small and green and fruits are purplish/greenish berries with 2-4 seeds.

What we use—Ripe fruits - fresh and dry, leaves, stems, flowers

What it does—*Fruit*—refrigerant, laxative, diuretic, haemostatic, aphrodisiac, antispasmodic, digestive

Leaves—diuretic, blood purifier, astrugent analysis

Flowers—expectorant, emmenagogue

How we use it—

In **anaemia**—Raisins with sugar or honey consumed twice a day conquers anaemia.

In **dry cough**—A decoction of grapes with honey is consumed twice a day for maximum relief.

In **thirst**—Dry grapes left overnight in warm water should be drunk the next morning to quench retention.

In **bleeding disorders**—Paste of raisins is licked with honey twice a day to arrest bleeding and cure associated anaemia.

As a **cosmetic**—Internal usage of grapes acts as a blood purifier and thereby improves complexion.

In **heart ailments**—Take an ounce of fresh grape juice everyday to tone your heart.

In **fainting**—To prevent fainting spells, give an ounce of fresh grape juice daily to the one affected. This improves blood circulation and reduces the incidence of fainting.

In **liver trouble**—Eating of fresh grapes is advised for a week. This will tone up sluggish liver.

42. Henna (Mehndi)

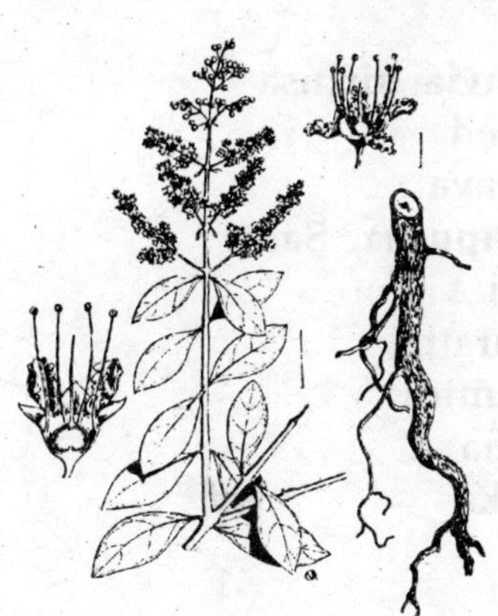

Also known as

Latin	:	**Lawsonia inermis**
English	:	**Henna**
Sanskrit	:	**Madayantika**
Hindi	:	**Mehndi**
Marathi	:	**Mehadi**
Tamil	:	**Mailanci, Marudani**
Telugu	:	**Goranta**
Malayalam	:	**Mailanchi**
Kannada	:	**Maurangi**

How it looks—It is a much branched woody shrub, its branches ending in spines, with white or rose-coloured fragrant flowers.

What we use—Root, leaves, flower, bark

What it does—*Roots*—diuretic, emmenagogue, refrigerant

Leaves—refrigerant, diuretic, emetic, expectorant, anti-inflammatory, liver tonic

Flowers—refrigerant, cardiotonic, febrifuge.

How we use it—

In **fungus and scabies**—In fungus affecting the crevices between the toes and fingers, apply a paste of henna leaves on the affected area and leave it on until the pack gets dry and cracks. Do this everyday until the infection is wiped out.

In **fainting and hysteria**—The peculiar smell of henna flowers has an invigorating effect in bouts of hysteria and fainting and reduces frequency of attacks.

In **sleeplessness**—Fitting a pillow with henna flowers before sleeping gives a restful slumber.

In **burns and scalds**—The decoction of the bark is a soothing agent when poured on the affected area.

In **headache**—Drink a cold infusion of the flowers twice a day to relieve headaches.

In **stomatitis**—Gargle frequently with a decoction of the leaves to soothe the oral ulcers.

In **gout**—The paste of the leaves is tied around the affected joints and left overnight to relieve burning sensation.

As a **blood purifier**—The decoction of henna flowers should be taken twice a day in skin infections and rashes to relieve itching and burning sensation.

43. Hogweed (Gadhahpurna)

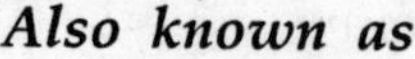

Also known as

Latin	:	**Boerrhavia diffusa**
English	:	**Hogweed**
Sanskrit	:	**Punarnava**
Hindi	:	**Gadhahpurna, Sant**
Marathi	:	**Ghetuli**
Tamil	:	**Mukkurattai**
Telugu	:	**Attamamidi**
Malayalam	:	**Tavilama**
Kannada	:	**Sanadika**

"Always praised" is the meaning of the Sanskrit name Punarnava

How it looks—It is a diffuse perennial herb with a stout root stock and many branches, typically seen with the onset of monsoon. The leaves are rounded or subcordate, whitish beneath and the flowers are pale pink, small and found in irregular clusters. The fruits are small, easily detachable and one-seeded.

What we use—Whole plant

What it does—It is cooling, anthelmintic, astringent, diuretic, aphrodisiac, cardiac stimulant, diaphoretic, emetic, expectorant, anti-inflammatory, febrifuge, laxative and tonic.

How we use it—

In **swellings**—Whether due to kidney or heart disease, it shows a remarkable decrease in swelling of the hands, feet, face or the entire body. Take a decoction of the roots or whole plant twice a day for increase in urine output and reduction of swelling.

As a **diuretic and aphrodisiac**—It removed obstruction to urination and is cooling to the system. It is therefore useful in cases of dysuria, urinary stones, burning urination apart from serving as a tonic to the urino-genital system.

In **hard unripe abscesses**—Make a decoction of the root of the white variety of hogweed and take twice a day to bring the abscess to ripening so as to facilitate draining of pus.

In **all skin disorders**—Make a paste of the root with the supernatant (floating) water on yogurt and apply on itching, discoloured or flaky skin patches to effect quick healing.

In **fevers**—Take a tsp of the dried and powdered hogweed roots with warm water or warm milk twice a day to bring down fevers, especially those accompanied with burning sensation.

In **eye disorders**—Hogweed can be used in a variety of ways for eye diseases just by pasting it with various substances and instilling a few drops in the eyes everyday.

1. In itching - with milk
2. In constant watering and other discharges - with honey
3. In unsteady vision and whitish patches on the cornea - with ghee
4. In immature cataract - with oil
5. In nightblindness - with rice wash

In **rheumatic disorders**—Especially in painful joints accompanied by swellings, hogweed can be used as a curry included in everyday diet. This removes constipation, promotes urination and reduces swelling and pain.

In **fevers**—Boil the powdered root of hogweed in milk and drink twice a day before your meals to reduce temperature and malaise.

44. Holy Basil (Tulsi)

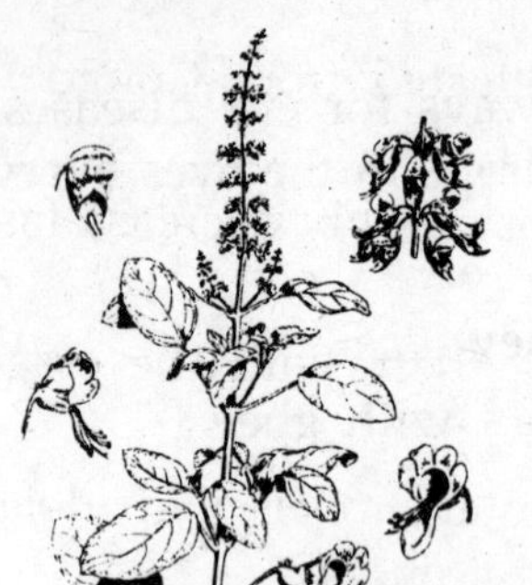

Also known as

Latin	**:**	**Ocimum basilicum**
English	**:**	**Holy Basil**
Sanskrit	**:**	**Tulasi, Surasah**
Hindi	**:**	**Kalatulsi**
Marathi	**:**	**Tulas**
Tamil	**:**	**Karuttulaci, Tulasi**
Telugu	**:**	**Tulasi**
Malayalam	**:**	**Krshnattulasi**
Kannada	**:**	**Karitulasi**

The sanskrit word "Tulasi" means "incomparable"

How it looks—It is an erect, aromatic, branching herb, with green or purplish leaves, white, green or pale purple leaves and oval black fruits.

What we use—whole plant

What it does—It is aromatic, thermogenic, anti-inflammatory antispasmodic, galactogogue, antibacterial, anti-emetic, insecticidal and antipyretic.

How we use it—

In **cough**—Drink the juice of the leaves of the black variety of tulsi with a tsp of honey thrice a day. Or you could chew the leaves from time to time.

In **irritation or pain in the throat**—Gargle with warm water in which tulsi leaves have been boiled, and drink the same, until relief is obtained.

In **night blindness**—Instill 2 drops of tulsi leaves in the eyes daily at bedtime.

In **insect sting or allergic rashes**—Drink tulsi juice in water and apply the fresh juice on the stung area to reduce inflammation. In skin infections too, the same procedure is highly beneficial.

In **hives or urticaria**—Take an infusion of tulsi leaves, neem leaves and fenugreek seeds with honey.

In **ear infections**—When there is pus in the ear and the ear emits a foul odour, a few drops of tulsi should be instilled in the ears to clear the pus and combat infection.

In **seasonal fevers**—Take tulsi leaf juice with pepper thrice a day to bring down the temperature and clearing the infection.

Modern Studies

1. Tulsi was found to increase humoral and cell-mediated immunity in experimental studies.
2. Antibacterial and antifungal effects of Rama Tulasi collected from Congo were demonstrated in experimental studies.
3. The leaf powder administrated to rats was shown to considerably decrease fasting blood sugar, total cholesterol and phospholipids.
4. Experimental studies on rats proved that administering them with the essential oil of tulsi helps correct behavioural reactions to stress.
5. Anti cataract activity of tulsi was observed in experimental models with delay in development of various stages of cataract on administration.

45. Indian Bdellium (Gugal)

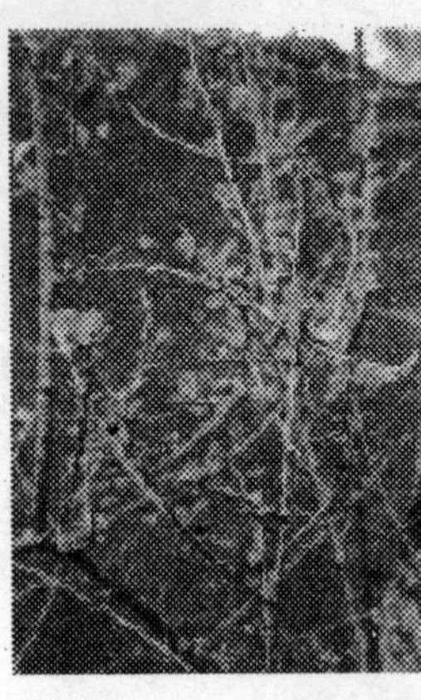

Also known as

Latin	**:**	**Commiphorahmukul**
English	**:**	**Indian bdellium tree**
Sanskrit	**:**	**Gugguluh**
Hindi	**:**	**Gugal**
Marathi	**:**	**Guggul**
Tamil	**:**	**Gukkulu**
Telugu	**:**	**Guggulam**
Malayalam	**:**	**Gulgulu**
Kannada	**:**	**Guggulu**

"That which protects from disease" is the meaning of the Sanskrit word Guggulu.

How it looks—It is a small armed tree with thorny branches and ash-coloured flaky bark. The young parts are glandular, and the leaves serrate in the upper parts and obovate otherwise. The flowers are small and brownish red with 8-10 stames and the fruits are drupes, red when ripe.

"Guggul" is the resinous gum, obtained from the bark. It is an irregular roundish glistening mass and is opaque, reddish brown when dry and aromatic.

What we use—*Gum resin*

What it does—It is aromatic, thermogenic, expectorant, digestive, anthelmintic, anti-inflammatory, anodyne, antiseptic, nervine tonic, demulcent, aphrodisiac, liver tonic, stimulant, antispasmodic, emmenagogue, haematinic, diuretic and rejuvenative.

How we use it—

In **injury**—Apply a mixture of myrrh and amhaldi over the wound to reduce pain and inflammation and quicken healing.

After **delivery**—Myrrh is highly indicated in women who have recently delivered, owing to its astringent, digestive, antiseptic and rejuvenative properties. Take a piece of myrrh and fry it in ghee (it swells like asafoetida). Mix it in a morsel of rice and give it to the woman who is recuperating after a delivery.

In **enlarged glands**—Guggulu or myrrh is used in a variety of combinations to reduce enlarged glands of the neck and benign tumours or to control inflammation of any sort. It may be fried in ghee and rolled into tiny pills and a pill may be taken twice a day.

In **tuberculosis**—Myrrh acts as antiseptic and anti-inflammatory and can be combined with asafoetida, ginger and some sugar to make small pills to be given in the early stage of tuberculosis to arrest progress of disease.

In **rheumatic swellings**—As a highly effective anti-inflammatory, myrrh resin can be given in joint swellings in combination with dry ginger and castor oil. Again, small pills are rolled out of the above mixture and one is given twice a day.

In **syphilis**—In late syphilis, when most other drugs fail, application of Guggulu internally and externally has been found to be useful.

In all the above preparations, myrrh resin which is over a year old is to be used for its enhanced medicinal value.

46. Indian Pennywort (Barami)

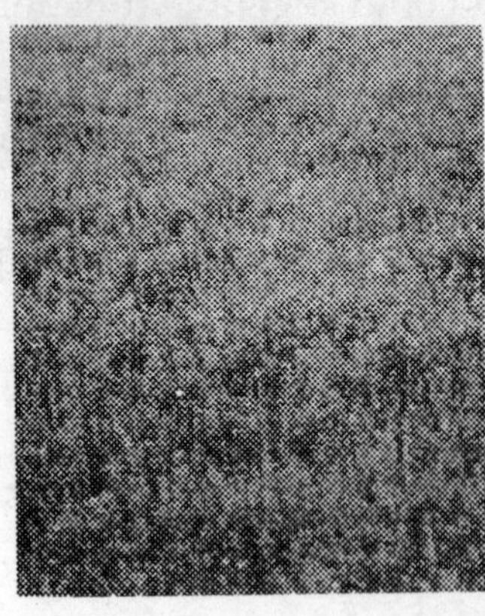

Also known as

Latin	:	Centella asiatica
English	:	Indian Pennywort
Sanskrit	:	Brahmi, Sarasvati
Hindi	:	Barami
Marathi	:	Brahmi
Tamil	:	Nirpirami
Telugu	:	Sambranichettu
Malayalam	:	Brahmi
Kannada	:	Nirbrahmi

Brahmi is now a widely publicised brain tonic, thanks to Ayurvedic companies highlighting its use in amentia, dementia, hysteria etc. It occupies a place of pride in the Ayurvedic materia medica owing to its multifarous applications.

How it looks—It is a slender herbaceous creeping perennial with heart shaped toothed leaves and pink flowers. The fruits are compressed sidewards with ridges.

What we use—Whole plant

What it does—It is cooling, cardiotonic, nervine tonic, stomachic, carminative, diuretic and febrifuge.

How we use it—

As a **brain tonic**—Chew 2-4 fresh green leaves along with some sugar on empty stomach every morning. This practice enhances memory and rectifies speech disorders apart from providing concentration and retention capacity.

In **mental disorders**—In schizo phrenia, hysteria and stress related psychoses, give a tsp of freshly expressed juice of the leaves with a tsp of honey everyday for calming the nerves and tranquilising the mind.

In **skin disorders**—Brahmi was reported to be an important adjuvant for treating obstinate skin disorders like psoriasis in clinical trials at Hyderabad. 80% of patients reported remarkable reduction of symptoms and signs within 40 days of treatment. Commercially avilable Brahmi vati was used.

In **respiratory disorders**—Brahmi is an important adjuvant in the treatment of all spasmodic respiratory disorders as it relaxes the airways and allows restful slumber.

Modern Studies

1. It was shown that bacosides from Brahmi extract augmented both cognitive function and mental retention capacity in experimental studies in Lucknow.
2. Relaxant effect of Brahmi extract in trachea, pulmonary artery and aorta was found in experimental studies on rabbits and guinea pig in Karachi.
3. Wound healing activity of ethanolic extract of brahmi was observed in normal and diabetic animals in Lucknow.

47. Khaskhas (khas-khas)

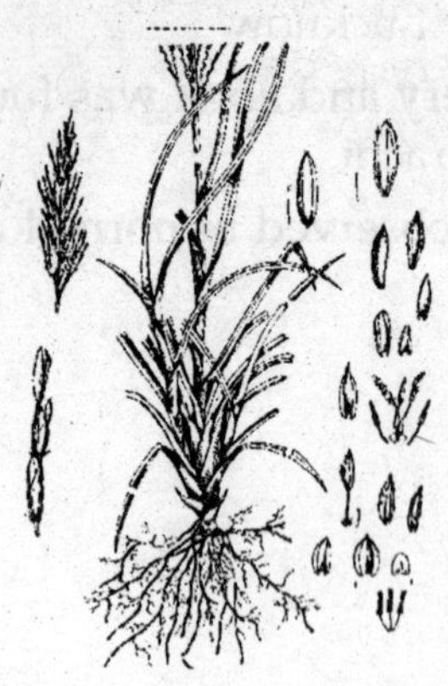

Also known as

Latin	**:**	**Vetiveria zizaniodes**
English	**:**	**Khaskhas**
Sanskrit	**:**	**Usirah**
Hindi	**:**	**Khas-khas**
Marathi	**:**	**Kalavala**
Tamil	**:**	**Vettiver**
Telugu	**:**	**Vettiverlu**
Malayalam	**:**	**Ramaccam**
Kannada	**:**	**Lamanci**

How it looks—It is a thick perennial grass, known for its pleasantly odoured roots and rhizomes. Its leaves are narrow and fruits oval.

What we use—Roots

What it does—It is a refrigerant, aromatic, digestive, carminative, anti-emetic, expectorant, diuretic, anthelmintic and antispasmodic.

How we use it—

In **bleeding disorders**—Equal parts of sandal and khaskhas powder are mixed in rice wash and taken along with sugar twice a day to arrest bleeding.

In **vomiting**—Water boiled in coriander seeds and khaskhas is an excellent remedy to suppress vomiting and nausea.

In **excessive perspiration**—The fine powder of khaskhas is rubbed over the body and left on for 15 minutes before a bath. This may also be done in measles to pacify the rashes.

In **fevers**—Steaming the body with water to which khaskhas is added promotes perspiration while bringing temperature down. Water boiled with khaskhas may be used as a drink in feverish conditions.

As a diuretic—In most conditions like painful urination, urinary stones and burning urine, drinking water boiled with khaskhas roots powder promotes urination, alleivates burning sensation and clears the passage of urine.

48. Land-calotrops (Gokhru)

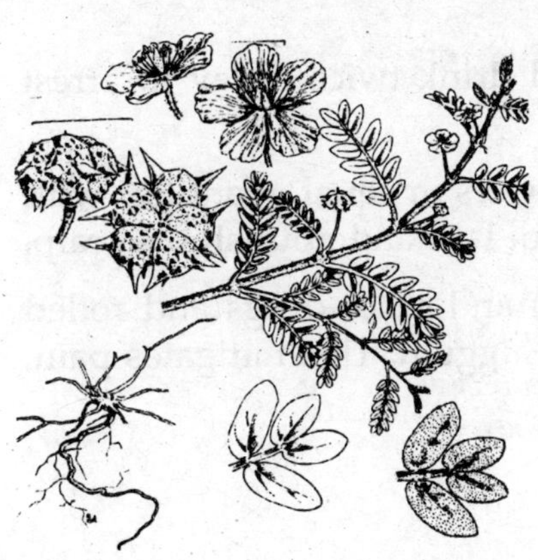

Also known as

Latin	:	**Tribulus terrestris**
English	:	**Land-calotrops**
Sanskrit	:	**Goshurah**
Hindi	:	**Gokhru**
Marathi	:	**Gogharu**
Tamil	:	**Nerinci**
Telugu	:	**Palleru**
Malayalam	:	**Nerinnil**
Kannada	:	**Negalu**

How it looks—It is an annual or perennial prostrate herb with many slender, spreading branches. The leaves are small, rounded at the base and shallowly pointed at the apex. The flowers are bright yellow and the fruits are 5-angled and woody separated into 5 segments. Each segment has 2 long stiff spines which are the characteristic features of the plant.

What we use—Whole plant

What it does—*Roots. & fruits*—cooling, diuretic, aphrodisiac, appetizer, digestive, anthelmentic, expectorant, anti-inflammatory, laxative, styptic, tonic.

Leaves—diuretic, aphrodisiac, anthelmentic, tonic.

Seeds—strengthening, astringent.

How we use it—

In **painful urination**—Boil a tsp of gokhru powder in milk and drink it to promote urination and reduce accompanying pain.

In **urinary stones**—Squeeze out the juice of the whole plant of gokhru and boil it in ghee until the juice evaporates completely. Take a tsp of this ghee with hot milk on empty stomach every morning.

Another method is to lick a tsp of powdered gokhru with honey and wash it down with goat milk. Follow this procedure for a week to break down urinary stones and expel them.

In **rheumatic joints**—Drink a decoction of gokhru and dry ginger every morning to reduce pain and improve digestion.

In **an aphrodisiac**—Boil the whole gokhru plant in milk and drink this milk at bedtime for an aphrodisiac effect.

In **consumption and wasting diseases**—Lick the powders of gokhru and ashwagandha with honey and wash it down with milk. This is rejuvenating, strengthening and improves resistance.

In **excessive bleeding**—Boil gokhru powder in milk and drink twice a day to arrest bleeding and build lost strength.

In **alopecia (bald patches)**—Paste gokhru and sesame flowers in equal quantities with honey and apply on the bald areas to stimulate regrowth of hair and nourish the scalp.

In **diabetes**—Gokhru is combined with Guggulu (myrrh) and other drugs and rolled into pills. This is available in the market as Gokshuradi Guggulu. This mitigates pain, swelling and such other conditions.

49. Lime (Nimbu)

Also known as

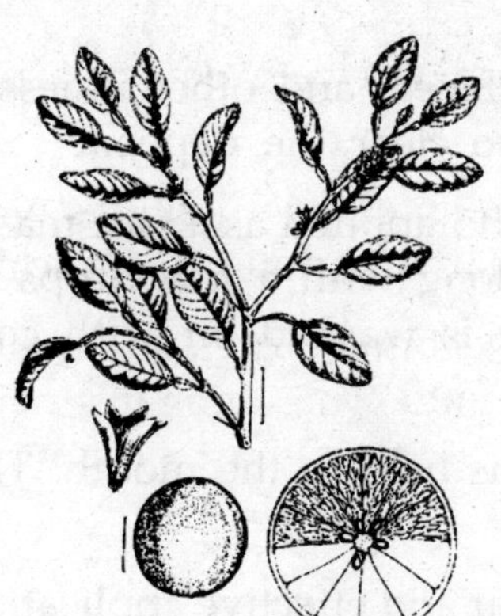

Latin	:	**Citrus limon**
English	:	**Lime**
Sanskrit	:	**Jambirah**
Hindi	:	**Nimbu**
Marathi	:	**Limbu**
Tamil	:	**Elumiccai**
Telugu	:	**Nimma**
Malayalam	:	**Uranarakam**
Kannada	:	**Limbe**

Lemon, like other citrus fruits like amla, orange and sweet orange owes its origin to China, and is best known for its high content of Vitamin C. Very few people know that it more importantly contains a substance called Vit. P which helps in the assimilation of Vit. C in the body. This places lemon and other fresh citrus fruits above all commercially available Vit. C tablets which do not serve the second purpose.

How it looks—It is a thorny shrub with spreading branches, aromatic leaves and white flowers. The fruits are large and spherical with pale acrid pulp and many seeds.

What we use—Fruits

What it does—It is digestive, carminative, stimulant, antiseptic, antiscorbutic, laxative, anthelmintic and anti-vertigo.

How we use it—

In **diarrhoea**—A mixture of onion juice and lime juice arrests mild diarrhoea, owing to its combination of antiseptic, astringent and nutritive properties.

In **bitter mouth**—Due to biliousness and indigestion, a bitter taste might persist in the mouth. Taking a glass of lime juice with a piece of ginger crushed into it is an ideal remedy.

> **General tip : Over sweetening the juice decreases its medicinal value. For best results, dilute it and take with a pinch of rock salt.**

In **piles**—Slit a small lime into two and sprinkle rock salt powder inside. Put this lime into the mouth and suck the juice slowly in. Do this regularly to heal pile masses.

In **cold**—Contrary to popular belief, lime is actually ideal in colds and fevers, unless you are specifically allergic to citrus fruits. Dilute lime juice with honey to drink is the best application in cases of common cold attacks.

In **chronic ear infections**—A few drops of filtered lime juice is instilled in the ears (This practice should be avoided in suspicion of a hole in the ear drum or such other ear damage.)

In **coated tongue**—This condition is common after chronic fevers and other illnesses due to indigestion. Rub a piece of lime over the tongue to clear the deposit.

In **oily skin**—Gramflour and honey are added to lime juice and applied as a face mask. In infected pimples, coconut milk is mixed in lime juice along with a few drops of rose petal juice and applied. After the application dries, it is washed off with cool water.

In **stomatitis and spongy gums**—About 10ml of lime juice is held in the mouth. The acid in lime juice kills any microbes causing infection.

In **dandruff**—Curd and lime juice on the scalp is a very popular and effective application against dandruff .Also, use a tsp of fresh lime juice in water for the last rinse of hair to remove stickiness.

In **obesity**—It is common knowledge that lime juice diluted and mixed with honey taken regularly, first thing in the morning is slimming apart from being helpful in clearing the skin.

To promote hair growth—Equal quantities of dried and powdered lime skin and the aerial roots of banyan are boiled in coconut oil. This oil used after filtering is good to stimulate hair growth.

In **patchy baldness**—Lime seeds and black pepper seeds are ground to a fine paste and applied to the bald patches to stimulate the scalp and induce growth of hair.

To **arrest bleeding**—Drink a glass of lime juice with a pinch of alum powder and sugar in it. In nasal bleeding, a few drops of lime juice instilled in the nose effects quick haemostasis.

In flatulence—It gives enough relief in excess gas formation when ½ lemon is squeezed in a cup of water and drunk 2/3 times a day. This will also give immediate relief in vertigo.

50. Liquorice/Mulhathi

Also known as

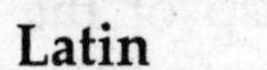

Latin	:	Glycyrrhiza glabra
English	:	Liquorice
Sanskrit	:	Yastimadhuh
Hindi	:	Jetimad, Mulhathi
Marathi	:	Jeshta madhu
Tamil	:	Atimaturam
Telugu	:	Atimadhuram
Malayalam	:	Irrattimadhuram
Kannada	:	Jesthamadhu

Caution—Liquorice is best avoided in pregnancy, heart and kidney disease and for prolonged periods.

How it looks—It is a tall, perennial undershrub, about 1 metre high, with violet bunched flowers and fibrous chocolate brown roots, which are yellow inside. The roots emit a sweet and pleasant odour.

What we use—Roots

What it does—It is a mild laxative, expectorant, aphrodisiac, intellect – promoting and haematinic

How we use it—

In **anaemia**—Make a decoction with a tsp of liquorice powder and water and drink twice a day with some honey.

In **bleeding per rectum**—Make a decoction of 2 tsp of liquorice root powder and water and take with honey twice a day.

In **blood vomiting**—Mix a tsp each of liquorice and sandal powder in milk and take twice a day.

In **flatulence**—Mix a tsp each of liquorice and sugar in water and drink from time to time.

In **sore throat**—Boil liquorice roots, tail pepper seeds and a few sugar candy crystals in milk and take an ounce thrice a day with honey to soothe throat irritation.

In **stomach ulcers**—The dry roots are soaked overnight in water and mixed with rice gruel and taken twice a day to heal gastric ulcers.

In **teeth cavities**—Powder liquorice sticks, pepper and ginger and fill the cavity with it. You can also use it as a tooth powder.

To increase breast milk secretion—A tsp of the powder should be consumed with milk and sugar twice a day by lactating mothers to increase production of milk.

In **epilepsy/fits**—Take a tsp of liquorice powder with the juice of ash pumpkin for 3 days consecutively.

In **pain in the bladder region**—Boil a tsp each of liquorice powder and raisins in milk and drink twice a day for relief from the pain.

In **emaciation in children**—Boil ½ tsp of liquorice in milk ,add some sugar and give the child this to drink twice a day to improve overall development.

For bone and joint problems—Take liquorice powder with milk to relieve joint aches, strengthen bones and for general good health.

In **corns**—When a corn starts sprouting, grind liquorice roots in mustard oil / gingelly oil and rub it in at bed time to soften the budding corn.

Modern Study

Anti-inflammatory effects of extracts of liquorice were demonstrated in experimental studies.

51. Lotus (Kamal)

Also known as

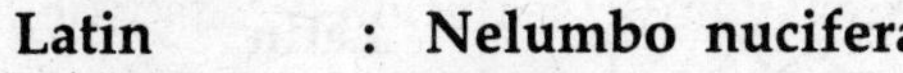

Latin	:	**Nelumbo nucifera**
English	:	**Lotus**
Sanskrit	:	**Padmam**
Hindi	:	**Kamal**
Marathi	:	**Kamala**
Tamil	:	**Tamarai**
Telugu	:	**Tamara**
Malayalam	:	**Tamara**
Kannada	:	**Kamala**

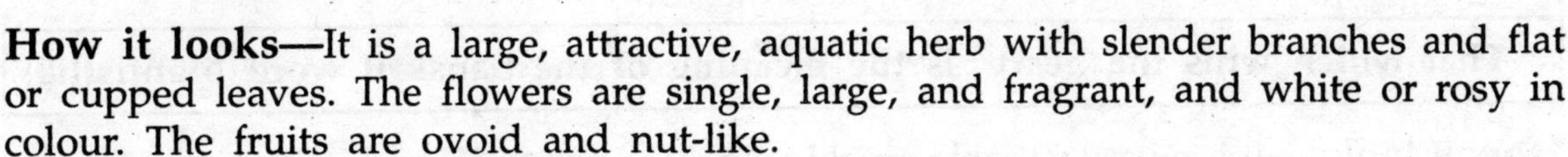

How it looks—It is a large, attractive, aquatic herb with slender branches and flat or cupped leaves. The flowers are single, large, and fragrant, and white or rosy in colour. The fruits are ovoid and nut-like.

What we use—Whole plant

What it does—It is astringent, cooling, emollient, diuretic, sudorific, antifungal and antipyretic, cardiotonic.

How we use it—

In **baldness**—Roots of lotus with aerial roots of banyan are dried and powdered. This powder is boiled in coconut oil and applied on the bald spots to stimulate hair growth.

In **painful urination**—Lotus petals and pink rose buds are made into a décoction to promote flow of urine and ease the pain.

As a **cardiac tonic**—White lotus petals are decocted and mixed in milk to make an effective cardiac tonic.

In **fever**—The roots and leaves of lotus which are available at all seasons can be made to a decoction to bring down fevers of all types.

52. Madder/Manjith

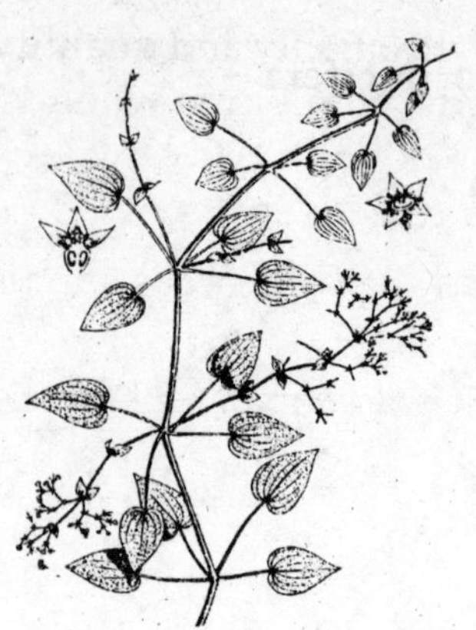

Also known as

Latin	:	**Rubia cordifolia**
English	:	**Madder root**
Sanskrit	:	**Manjistha, Yojanavalli**
Hindi	:	**Manjith**
Marathi	:	**Manjistha**
Tamil	:	**Sevvalli**
Telugu	:	**Tamravalli**
Malayalam	:	**Mancatti**
Kannada	:	**Manjistha**

"That which wins the heart" is the meaning of the Sanskrit word Manjistha

How it looks—It is a very variable, prickly climbing perennial herb with long, smooth, reddish cylindrical roots and 4-angled rough stems. The leaves are rounded or slightly heart shaped and the flowers are white green, yellowish or reddish and sweet-scented. The fruits are purplish black when ripe with 2 seeds.

What we use—Roots

What it does—It is bitter, astringent, thermogenic, anti-inflammatory, anodyne, antiseptic, digestive, carminative, anthelmentic, antidysenteric, emmenagogue, diuretic, galactopurifier, alterant, febrifuge and tonic.

How we use it—

As a **blood purifier**—The decoction of the roots of madder is indicated in all skin disorders like fungal infections eczema, psoriasis and discolourations .Even in diabetic wounds, the feet should be immersed in the cooled decoction of madder every day for rapid healing. This is due to the antiseptic and astringent properties of madder.

As a **cosmetic**—In blackened patches over the face, long-term use of madder and milk as a face pack ensures lightening of patches and normal colouration of skin.

In **scanty menses**—Drink a decoction of madder roots for an entire menstrual cycle everyday to correct anaemia if any and establish a healthy flow of menstrual blood.

In **sore throat**—For reviving an over used throat, drink hot milk with a tsp of madder root powder and some sugar in it.

In **scanty urination**—Being diuretic, a decoction of sandal or khaskhas roots along with madder ensures free flow of urination.

In **swellings**—For the same reason, it removes excess fluid from the body through urine and aids reduction of swelling.

In **bleeding disorders**—As it is a haematinic and improves both the quality and quantity of blood, it is highly indicated in excessive bleeding from any orifice and from wounds.

Modern Studies

1. The aqueous extract of madder exhibited antibacterial effect on staphylococcus aureus (gram positive) in experimental studies.
2. The methanolic extracts exhibited anticancer activity which was comparable to 5–fluoruracil.

53. Malabar Nut (Adusa)

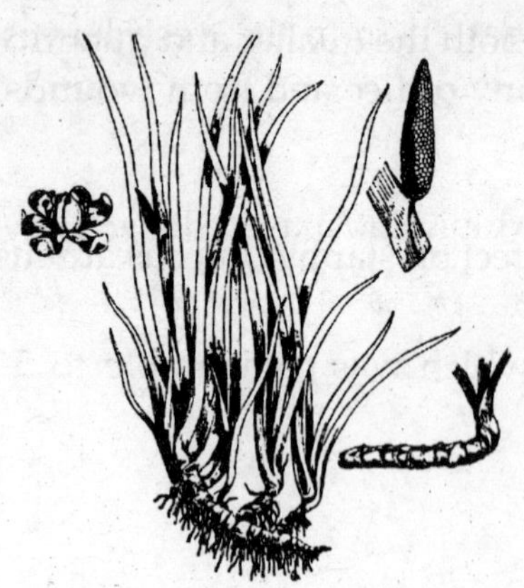

Also known as

Latin	:	Adhatoda Vasika
English	:	Malabar Nut tree
Sanskrit	:	Vasa
Hindi	:	Adusa
Marathi	:	Adulasa
Tamil	:	Adutota
Telugu	:	Addasaramu
Malayalam	:	Atalotakam
Kannada	:	Sanna

Adhatoda got its name from the south, "Aduthoda" meaning, "that which a goat does not touch" owing to its bitter taste.

How it looks—It is a large, glabrous shrub, with opposite, short-petioled leaves and short flower heads. The fruits are capsules.

What we use—Whole plant

What it does—It is bitter, astringent, refrigerant, expectorant, diuretic, antispasmodic, febrifuge, styptic depurative and tonic.

How we use it—

Bleeding disorders—It is the drug of choice in bleeding of any kind – dysentery, menorrhagia, metrorrhagia, bleeding piles, or bleeding from wounds.

Squeeze the juice out of steamed fresh leaves and drink an ounce of the juice, sweetened with honey, twice a day.

In **chronic coughs**—In all kinds of cough, eating a tsp of a confectionery made of the whole vasa plant, pepper, sugar, ghee and honey is highly relieving. Being anti spasmodic it soothes bronchial spasms and is widely used in asthmatic conditions.

In **tuberculosis**—The juice of the leaves is used to liquify sputum. "Gulkand" is a preparation made out of vasa flowers, used to treat tuberculosis.

The readymade market preparation vasarishta, a liquid is also beneficial in doses of 20ml twice a day after meals.

Painful joints—Apply a poultice of the slightly warmed leaves on fresh wounds, rheumatic joints and swellings.

In **skin disorders**—Especially in itching skin conditions like scabies, eczema, the decoction of the leaves is used internally and to sprinkle on the lesions.

In **worm infestations**—Take a quarter cup of the juice expressed from the fresh leaves twice a day to dislodge and expel intestinal worms.

Modern Study

Vascine, an alkaloid extracted from vasaka was shown to exhibit antispasmodic activity in experimental studies on rats.

54. Mango (Aam)

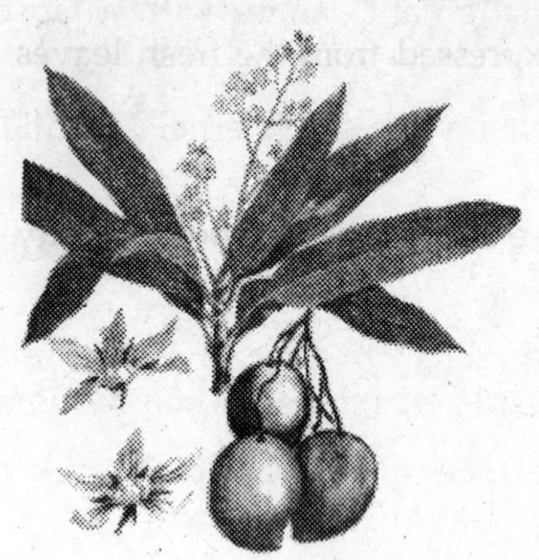

Also known as

Latin	**:**	**Mangifera Indica**
English	**:**	**Mango**
Sanskrit	**:**	**Amrah**
Hindi	**:**	**Aam**
Marathi	**:**	**Amba**
Tamil	**:**	**Mamaram**
Telugu	**:**	**Mamidi**
Malayalam	**:**	**Mavu**
Kannada	**:**	**Mavu**

Mango is undoubtedly the most loved and praised fruit, indigenous to India. Whether in popularity, nutritive value, production value or versatility in use, it holds a leading edge over all other fruits. In fact, the mango has so much been identified with India that it has been repeated in the paisley design prominently featuring in fabrics, jewellery and embroidery denoting Indian culture.

It has been mentioned several times in ancient epics such as the Ramayana, the Mahabharata, the Meghadoota by Kalidasa and in works of other authors such as Panini and Amara Sinha. It holds great sentimental value by being an integral part of all auspicious occasions, the flowers being used in Saraswati Pooja and the leaves serving as decorative festoons at thresholds, probably owing to their anti-bacterial activity.

Nutritive value—It is an outstanding source of vitmin A and a good source of vitamin c, apart from the usual content of minerals mainly iron, calcium, phosphorous—5,000 IU, consist of 20% of total soluble solids (sugars)

How it looks—It is a large, spreading evergreen tree with small reddish or yellowish—green flowers, and large fleshy fruits containing a hard fibrous seed.

What we use—Roots bark, leaves, flowers, fruits, seed kernel.

What it does—*Roots & bark*—astringent, styptic, anti-inflammatory

Leaves—astringent, refrigerant, styptic

Flowers—astringent, refrigerant, styptic, haematinic

Fruits—digestive, carminative, refrigerant, antifungal

Seed Kernel—anthelmintic, constipating, styptic and uterine tonic

How we use it—

In **vomiting**—Cold infusion of the tender leaves of mango and jamun with a tsp of honey serves to suppress vomiting and nausea.

In **bleeding from the nose**—About 3-4 drops of the juice of the seed kernel , instilled in the nostrils arrests the bleeding immediately.

In **splenomegaly**—(enlargement of spleen) Make a habit of drinking the juice of a ripe mango with a tablespoon of honey everyday.

In **blood in motions**—A few pieces of the bark of the mango tree are boiled in milk and given along with some honey twice a day until blood stops appearing in motions.

In **dandruff**—Make an application of the bark of the mango tree pasted in milk or just plain water, on the head for a few week to rid yourself of dandruff.

In **diarrhoea**—During its season, collect mango seeds, dry them in the shade, powder and sieve, and store the powder for such emergencies as diarrhoea. Make small balls of this powder with jaggery in case of diarrhoea and take one ball thrice a day. The seed powder alone is useful in piles.

In **boils**—An application of the mango bark paste on boils just coming up, quickly suppresses them. Internally, an infusion made from the raw mango pulp squeezed into water acts as an astringent. Raw mango is also rich in ascorbic acid or vitamin C, which quickens healing.

In **insect stings**—To prevent inflammation apply the juice of the mango leaf on the stung area, or even the milk oozing from a plucked stalk of the leaf.

Mango in any form arrests bleeding. The bark, roots, leaves, fruit, flower and leaves - all act as styptic agents.

In **diabetes**—Though diabetics cannot enjoy mango fruits; they may find its very tender leaves to be an answer to their plight. The leaves are dried, powdered and stored. Half a tsp of this powder should be taken twice a day. Even the infusion of the fresh leaves is useful in diabetes.

Panna - A Summer Coolant

Boil an unripe mango in 250ml water and filter the water. Add some powdered cumin, rock salt and palm candy to make a sweet cooling beverage for those hot days.

In **sunstroke**—A drink made from boiled, unripe mango with salt and sugar is a wonderful remedy for sunstroke.

55. Mesua (Nagakesar)

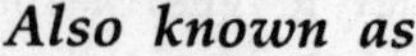

Also known as

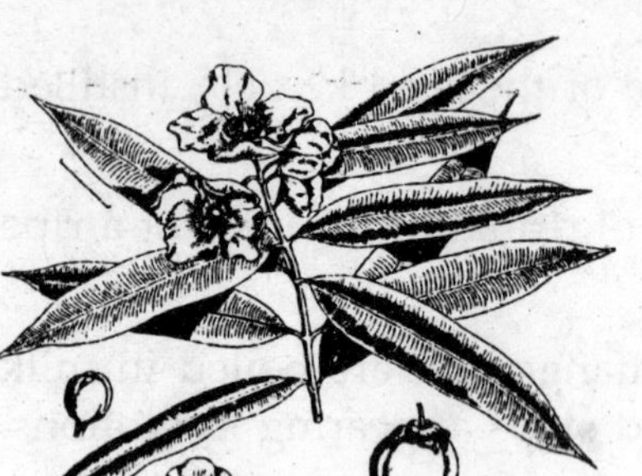

Latin	:	**Mesua ferrea**
English	:	**Mesua, Iron-wood tree**
Sanskrit	:	**Nagakesarah, Punnaga**
Hindi	:	**Nagakesar**
Marathi	:	**Nagakeshar**
Tamil	:	**Nagappu**
Telugu	:	**Nagakesaramu**
Malayalam	:	**Nagappuvu**
Kannada	:	**Nagasampige**

"Best among trees" is the meaning of the Sanskrit name Punnaga.

How it looks—It is a medium sized to large, evergreen tree with sharp edge simple leaves and brown flaky bark. The flowers are white, fragrant with numerous stamens which are golden yellow in colour and very short. The fruits are ovoid with 1-4 angular, smooth seeds.

What we use—Flowers, oil

What it does—It is astringent, mildly heating, anodyne, sudorific, digestive, carminative, anthelmintic, diuretic, haemostatic, aphrodisiac, cardiotonic and febrifuge.

How we use it—

In **bleeding piles and dysentery**—Best known for its haemostatic property, the powder of the flowers is given with butter and sugar twice a day until bleeding stops.

In **leucorhhoea**—Pasted flowers of mesua with curd is given in doses of 2 tsp twice a day until white discharge disappears. This treatment should be followed by a diet of rice and buttermilk.

In **dysuria**—A decoction of the flowers of mesua should be taken sweetened with sugar in conditions such as painful or burning urination, difficult urination or blood in urine.

In **excessive menstrual bleeding**—A tsp of the powder mixed in buttermilk is a good remedy to arrest excessive bleeding per vagina, or bleeding of any sort.

In **skin disorders**—In itching, oozing and black of reddish discolouration of skin, the seed oil of mesua serves as a good external application and normalizes skin. It is therefore a chief component of many a cosmetic preparation.

In **fevers**—Mesua promotes perspiration and thereby brings down temperature. For this purpose, the bark powder is generally used to prepare a decoction .

In **gouty joints**—The seed oil makes an excellent soothing external application and also appeases associated pain and burning sensation.

Modern Study

The phenolic constituents of the seed oil have been shown to possess powerful anti-asthmatic effects in experimental studies.

56. Mustard (Rayi)

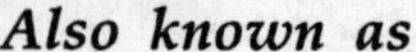

Also known as

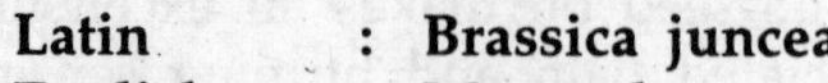

Latin	:	Brassica juncea
English	:	Mustard
Sanskrit	:	Sharshapa
Hindi	:	Rayi
Marathi	:	Mohari
Tamil	:	Katugu
Telugu	:	Avalu
Malayalam	:	Katuku
Kannada	:	Sasive

How it looks—It is a glabrous annual with a few bristles at the base and leaves which are broad and coarsely dentate at the edges. The flowers are yellow and fruits are pod like breaking from below upwards with many seeds.

What we use—Seeds, oil

What it does—It is thermogenic, anodyne, anti-inflammatory, carminative, digestive, anthelmintic, sudorific and tonic.

How we use it—

In **asthma**—During an attack, massage warm mustard oil to which a little camphor is added over the chest and back. This liquidates phlegm and clear the airways. You could also roast a lemon packed in mud on fire and squeeze the warm lemon (after breaking the mud pack) in some warm mustard oil. Use this mixture to massage over the chest, back and neck to loosen and expectorate obstructing phlegm.

In **swollen and painful joints**—To reduce stiffness and pain in joints, apply a mixture of mustard oil and camphor and massage lightly. It acts as a counter irritant and improves blood circulation.

In a **stiff neck**—It is a common practice to apply mustard oil on a stiff neck and run a rolling pin over on the neck to ease the stiffness and pain.

In **leg cramps**—Massage the feet and legs with warm mustard oil prepared by adding a few pieces of ginger, some pepper powder and cumin seeds; this relieves the tired legs and refreshes the muscles.

In **headache**—Applying a paste of mustard over the temples mixed in oil for a heavy head serves as a counter irritant and relieves heaviness and congestion in the head.

57. Margosa (Neem)

Also known as

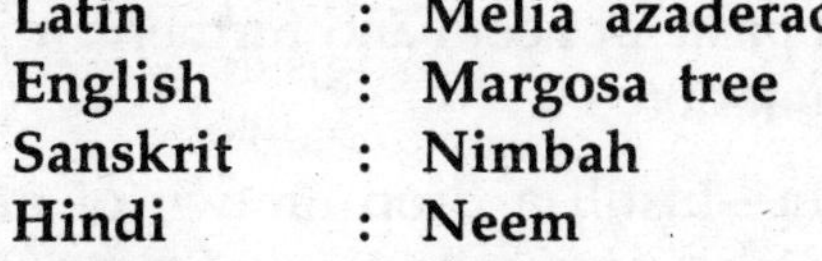

Latin	:	Melia azaderach
English	:	Margosa tree
Sanskrit	:	Nimbah
Hindi	:	Neem
Marathi	:	Nimba
Tamil	:	Vempu, Veppai
Telugu	:	Kondavepa
Malayalam	:	Veppu
Kannada	:	Turagavepu

Neem is probably one of the oldest and most widely used medicinal plants in India. It has been an inherent part of traditional festivals like "Ugadi", the Telugu new year's day, where a chutney is made of the flowers. It is the most recognised and medicinally valued tree in India

How it looks—It is a moderate sized deciduous tree with a cylindrical dark grey trunk with shallow furrowed bark. The leaves are serrated and the flowers are lilac, fragrant with a prominent staminal tube. The fruits are globose and 4-seeded and turn yellow when ripe.

What we use—Roots, leaves, seeds, flowers.

What it does—*Roots*—bitter, astringent, anodyne, depurative, antiseptic, anthelmintic, constipating, expectorant, urinary astringent, emmenagogue, tonic.

Leaves—astringent, expectorant, vermicidal, diuretic, emmenagogue, stomachic.

Seeds—expectorant, anthelmintic, aphrodisiac

Flowers—astringent, refrigerant, stomachic, vermifuge, diuretic, emmenagogue.

How we use it—

In **intestinal parasites**—Take about 10 drops of neem oil in a glass of your favourite beverage to get rid of worms and other infestations.

You could also use the fresh leaf juice of neems with a pinch of rock salt for the same effect.

In **eruptive fevers**—Drink neem decoction from time to time in chicken pox and measles to get rid of vesicles and stroke the itching lesions with neem leaves. Making a bed of neem leaves is a very useful idea. When the lesions dry up, grind turmeric rhizome and neem leaves and paste it on the healing boils to hasten recovery and as a disinfectant. Use neem – boiled water to take bath in.

In **mumps**—Make a paste of neem and turmeric to apply on the swellings for reduction of pain and inflammation.

In **ear inflammation**—Instill a drop or two of neem oil in the painful ear to bring down infection and dry any collection of pus and wax.

In **itching vagina**—Wash the area with warm water and then with neem decoction. This helps to immediately relieve itching and keeps the area germ-free.

Teeth care—Neem twigs as toothbrushes have been popular for centuries. They act by virtue of their natural astringent, antiseptic and anthelmintic activities to keep the oral cavity clear of gum and tooth infections, pyorrhoea and ulcers.

In **skin infection**—The best known use of neem is its property of keeping the skin clear and free of infections, which is why neem-boiled water was used for bath until recent times.

The internal use of neem decoction too helps control even obstinate skin diseases like leprosy and psoriasis, while curing scabies, urticaria, allergic rashes and the like.

Using neem oil for external application is a surefire remedy for wet, oozing lesions and accompanying inflammation and itching.

In **jaundice**—Drink the diluted juice of the tender neem leaves with a tsp of honey to flush out toxins in liver disorders.

Modern Studies

Recent experimental studies in Delhi on leaf extracts of neem showed its immunopotentiating and adaptogenic effects in mice.

1. Anti hyperglycemic activity of neem leaf extract was observed in experimental studies on non-insulin dependent diabetes mellitus – induced rats.
2. Antifertility effects of aqueous and steroidal extract of neem leaf were observed in an experimental study in West Indies.
3. Immunomodulatory effects of NIM-76, a volatile fraction of neem oil were found in experimental studies in Delhi.
4. Anti diabetic and antihyperlipemic effects of neem seed powder were observed in experimental studies in Baroda.

58. Nutmeg (Jayphal)

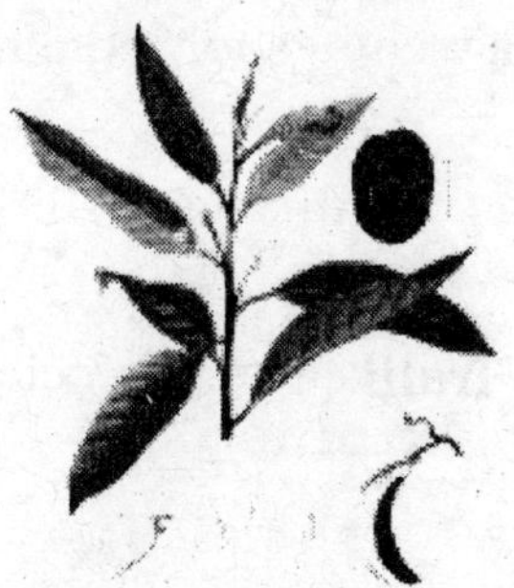

Also known as

Latin	:	**Myrstica fragrans**
English	:	**Nutmeg tree**
Sanskrit	:	**Jati, Jatiphalah**
Hindi	:	**Jaykapet, Jayphal**
Marathi	:	**Jatphal**
Tamil	:	**Jastimaram, Jatikkai**
Telugu	:	**Jajikaya**
Malayalam	:	**Jatikka**
Kannada	:	**Jajikayi**

How it looks—it is a moderate sized aromatic, evergreen tree with creamy yellow fragrant flowers and yellow fruits which split on maturity. The seeds are oval with yellowish red arils.

What it does—It is anti-inflammatory, aphrodisiac, anthelmintic, expectorant, digestive and carminative.

How we use it—

In **thirst & vomiting**—A cold infusion of nutmeg quenches thirst and suppresses nausea and vomiting.

In **black discolourations**—Paste nutmeg with some water and apply on the face to rid yourself of spots and discolorations. This paste is effective in healing cracked soles too.

In **indigestion**—The volatile oils present in nutmeg are digestive and carminative, and thereby a decoction of nutmeg is highly beneficial in such conditions.

In **headache**—As a topical application in headache, the paste of nutmeg provides quick relief.

In **arthritis**—The oil of nutmeg is mixed with mustard oil and applied on painful joints for relief. Even a paste of nutmeg can be applied in the absence of oil.

In **diarrhoea**—The decoction of the heartwood of nutmeg is useful in arresting diarrhoea.

In **burning eyes**—Nutmeg is rich in fats and volatile oils and so is used for its beneficial effects on the eyes. Paste nutmeg in milk and apply all around the eyes and over the eyelids for its cooling effects.

Modern Study

Experimental studies on an extract of nutmeg showed that it significantly lowers total cholesterol levels in the heart.

Warning

Eating too much nutmeg produces narcotic effect causing delirium and convulsions.

59. Onion (Pyaz)

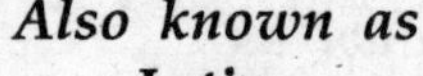

Also known as

Latin	:	Allium cepa
English	:	Onion
Sanskrit	:	Palandu
Hindi	:	Pyaz
Marathi	:	Kanda
Tamil	:	Venkayam, Trulli
Telugu	:	Ullipaya
Malayalam	:	Cuvannulli
Kannada	:	Nirulli

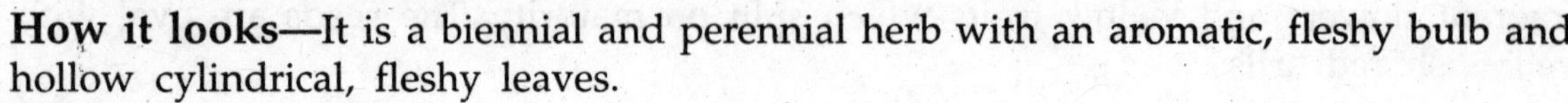

How it looks—It is a biennial and perennial herb with an aromatic, fleshy bulb and hollow cylindrical, fleshy leaves.

What we use—Bulbs

What it does—It is aromatic, thermogenic, antibacterial, aphrodisiac, emmenagogue, expectorant, carminative and diuretic

How we use it—

In **bleeding from nose**—Instilling a few drops of onion juice in the nose will arrest the bleeding.

In **bleeding piles**—Using onions in the diet is beneficial in piles. White onions shredded and fried in ghee are mixed with rice and eaten.

In **hiccups & breathing disorders**—A few drops of onion juice are instilled in the nostrils until relief is obtained.

In **eruptive fevers**—As a prophylactic for small pox, chicken pox and measles, a plateful of sliced onions is kept near the bed to disinfect the air.

In **conjunctivitis**—White onion juice is extracted fresh and a few drops instilled in the eyes to subside inflammation and speeden recovery.

In **fungal infection and scabies**—Onion juice is taken internally and the lesions are also rubbed with a combination of onion and betel juice.

In **septic pimples**—Remove the outermost scale of a juicy onion and leave it in salt solution for a few hours and then grate it. Rub the onion juice on the face and apply the gratings on the septic spots to soften and smoothen the skin.

After delivery—Make a decoction of a handful of peeled white onions, a tablespoonful of cumin seeds and a handful of brahmi leaves, and give this daily to restore normalcy to the body of a woman who has recently delivered.

To increase virility—Pink onions are grated and fried in ghee to make an excellent source of sexual vitality. A tsp of this is taken everyday.

As a **general tonic**—Including onions in plenty in the diet not only cures infections but improves resistance to fight infections.

In **severe diarrhoea**—A glass of equal quantities of onion juice and lime juice thrice a day can be tried before resorting to powerful drugs.

60. Papaya (Pappita)

Also known as

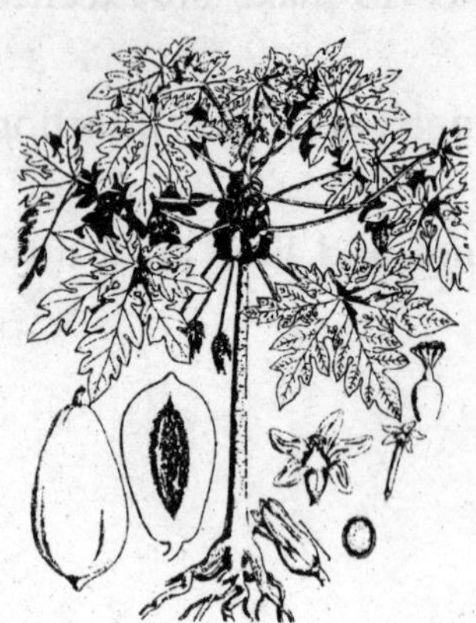

Latin	:	**Carica papaya**
English	:	**Papaw tree, papaya**
Sanskrit	:	**Erandakarkati**
Hindi	:	**Pappita**
Marathi	:	**Papai**
Tamil	:	**Pappali**
Telugu	:	**Boppayi**
Malayalam	:	**Pappali**
Kannada	:	**Peragi, Piranji**

How it looks—It is a small, soft wooded, milk-oozing tree with typical palm like leaves, and yellow cylindrical fruits.

What we use—Fruits, latex

What it does—It is thermogenic, anodyne, aphrodisiac, stomachic, digestive, carminative, diuretic, anthelmintic, anti-haemorrhoidal & cardio-tonic.

How we use it—

In **constipation**—Take a glass of papaya juice with breakfast for good digestion and soft stools.

In **chronic ulcers on skin**—Mix some butter in the juice of a papaya and apply for quick drying and healing of long-standing ulcers.

In **corns and warts**—Touch the hardened skin of the corn/wart with the milky juice oozing from the papaya leaf tip to soften it.

In **delayed periods**—Eat the green unripe papaya in case of delayed periods, to bring on menstrual flow. Its abortifacient qualities are also well known.

As a **diet**—Papaya is one fruit which despite its sweetness is not contra-indicated in diabetes. It is not only nutritious,but is also a digestive and relieves flatulence.

In **respiratory disorders**—The latex is useful in respiratory disorders like cough, bronchitis and breathlessness.

As a **cosmetic**—The dried latex and fruit pulp is useful as an ingredient in face masks and to get rid of acne and boils on the face.

In **enlargement of liver and spleen**—The pectin, citric acid, malic acid and other vitamins make the papaya fruit highly indicated in all digestive disorders and in hepatomegaly and splenomegaly.

Modern Study

The antifertility activity of the alcoholic extract of papaya seeds was noted in experimental studies in Brazil. This suggests that the seed extract can be utilized to develop safe contraceptives.

61. Peepal (Pippal)

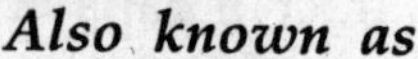

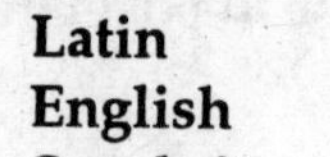

Also known as

Latin : Ficus religiosa
English : Peepal tree
Sanskrit : Ashathhah, Pippalah
Hindi : Pippal
Marathi : Pimpal
Tamil : Arasu
Telugu : Ravi
Malayalam : Arayal
Kannada : Aswaththa

How it looks—It is a large, woody tree with few or no aerial roots and drooping branchlets. The leaves are shining and ornate and rustle in the wind typically. The bark is ash-coloured with thin membranous flakes and patches.

What we use—Bark, leaves, tender shoots, fruits, seeds.

What it does—*Bark*—astringent, cooling, aphrodisiac
Fruits—laxative, digestive
Leaves and Tender shoots—purgative
Seeds—refrigerant, laxative.

How we use it—

In **inflammation and burns**—A paste of the powdered bark is a good absorbent for inflammatory swellings and burns.

'Peepal' is one of the drugs most used as an antiseptic and is beneficial in the treatment of ulcers. It relives burning sensation and reduces accumulated fat in the obesity.

In **diseases of uterus and vagina**, a deccoction of the bark is highly useful.

In **Gouty arthritis**—Peepal bark decoction in the dose of 15ml twice a day with equal quantity of water is used with honey.

In **gouty arthritis**—The tender leaves of peepal are made into a decoction and poured on the joints to relieve pain.

For **vigour and vitality**—The fruit of root, bark, and tender shoots are boiled with milk and taken internally with sugar and honey in doses of 15ml twice a day for an aphrodisiac effect.

Fractures: The barks of the peepal, palaash,and banyan trees are very useful in bandaging broken bones as soft but strong splints.

In **sterility in women**—A plant growing in peepal tree, popularly known as BADANIKA is boiled with milk and given internally in the suitable dosage and form. It helps in establishing pregnancy.

In **vomiting**—Vomiting can be controlled effectively by the ash of the bark well mixed in water. It should be allowed to settle down. This supernatant fluid is filtered and given repeatedly in severe vomiting.

Ulcers in the mouth: Fine powder of peepal bark should be applied, well-mixed in honey inside the oral cavity regularly. This effectively checks ulcers within 10 to 12 days time.

Modern Study

The aqueous extract of the bark exhibited antibacterial activity against Staphylococcus aureus and Escherichia coli.

62. Black Pepper (Kalimirch)

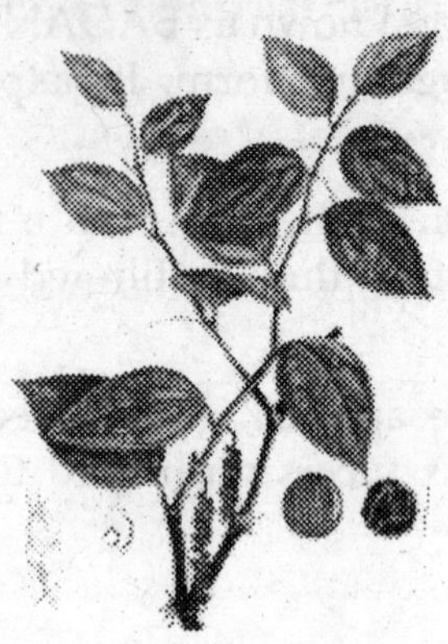

Also known as

Latin	**:**	**Piper nigrum**
English	**:**	**Black Pepper**
Sanskrit	**:**	**Maricam**
Hindi	**:**	**Kalimirch**
Marathi	**:**	**Mirch**
Tamil	**:**	**Milaku**
Telugu	**:**	**Miriyalu**
Malayalam	**:**	**Kurumulaku**
Kannada	**:**	**Ollimonasu**

The Sanskrit word "maricha" for pepper means—"that which destroys toxins"

How it looks—It is a stout climbing perennial with roots at the nodes. The leaves are heart shaped and the flowers spiky and very small. The fruits are globose and one-seeded and appear bright red when ripe with rounded seeds.

What we use—Fruits

What it does—It is anthelmintic, carminative, aphrodisiac, emmenagogue, stimulant, digestive, diuretic and alterant.

How we use it—

In **cough**—Powdered pepper with honey, ghee and saunph is licked to relieve from all kinds of cough.

In **hysteria**—Black pepper with bach is taken to soothe nerves in cases of hysteria.

In **diarrhoea**—1 tsp of fine powder of pepper should be taken with water to arrest diarrhoeas of even very chronic nature.

Lack of appetite and cough—Black pepper powder is gently roasted in a pan, powdered and mixed in molten jaggery. This preparation is rolled into tiny pills and allowed to become firm on cooling and stored. Pill should be taken twice a day to stimulate appetite.

In **indigestion**—Pepper powder mixed in butter milk, is a good digestive.

In **colds**—To relieve from colds , pepper made into a "rasam" with tamarind is a popular remedy. To a tsp of hot ghee, ½ tsp of black pepper powder is added, to which dilute tamarind water is added and boiled for a few minutes. Some coriander leaves may be added in the end for additional effect. The patient experiences the effect of fomentation while taking this "Rasam" and thereby nasal blockage is relieved.

In **pus in gums**—Finely powdered pepper and salt is massaged over the gums to relieve inflammation.

In **painful joints**—Pepper, cumin and ginger boiled in mustard oil is an effective massage oil to apply on painful joints.

In **stammering**—Mix almond without seed coat and black pepper in equal amount. Make a paste, add honey, take it in the morning for a month.

Modern Studies

1. Pepper has been shown to enhance bioavailability in experimental studies.
2. Pepper was part of an ayurvedic formulation found effective against dental diseases in a study conducted at Udaipur.

63. Picrorhiza (Kutki)

Also known as

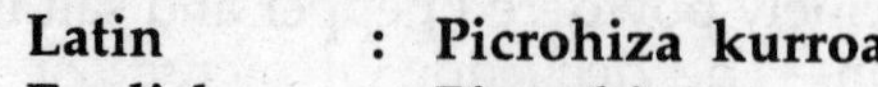

Latin : Picrohiza kurroa
English : Picrorhiza
Sanskrit : Katukarohini
Hindi : Kutki
Marathi : katuka
Tamil : Katugarohini
Telugu : Katki
Malayalam : Katukarohini
Kannada : Katukarohini

> **"That which envelopes diseases" is the meaning of the Sanskrit name 'katuki'.**

How it looks—It is a small, hairy, perennial herb, with a long woody root stock. The leaves are long with serrated edges and the flowers are white or bluish located terminally on long racemes, the fruits are ovoid capsules.

The dried rhizome is deep greyish brown, cylindrical and wrinkled longitudinally.

What we use—The dried rhizome

What it does—The rhizomes are cooling, laxative, digestive, carminative, anthelmintic, anti-inflammatory, galacto purifier, expectorant and anti-pyretic.

How we use it—

In **liver disorders** :Picrorhiza is an excellent liver protective and has been effective in cases of jaundice and chronic malaria where even quinine has failed. Make a decoction of equal quantifies of picrorhiza, and chirata and drink twice a day.

In **chronic malaria**—Make a decoction of equal quantities of pircrorhiza, chirata, harad fruit and sonamukhi leaves with sufficient quantity of jaggery and raisins in it. Filter and drink everyday. This decoction acts as a mild laxative and completely detoxifies the body. (you could omit the sonamukhi leaves in children)

In **anaemia**—Drink a decoction of the rhizome of picrorhiza for a few weeks to replenish last blood and as rejuvenator. This is especially useful in anaemia due to excessive bleeding from any orifice.

In **disorder of breastmilk**—Its decoction is highly beneficial in recently delivered women as it establishes free flow of breastmilk and removes associated disorders.

In **respiratory allergies**—Picroliv, present in picrorhiza is a known immunomodulator, making it a sought after home remedy in bronchitis, asthma and sinusitis. As above, a decoction of the rhizome is used.

In **worm infestation**—The decoction of picrorhiza is mild enough to be given as a deworming medicine even to children.

In **indigestion**—Its natural liver-protective property make picrorhiza an ideal choice in all cases of indigestion. It also removes associated loss of taste sensation.

Modern Studies

1. Anti-allergic activity of picroliv, a standardised fraction isolated from picrorhiza kurroa was demonstrated in experimental studies on guinea pig in Lucknow.
2. Anti oxidant and lipid metabolism-regulating activity of picroliv was established in studies in Lucknow.
3. Hepato protective activity of picrorin was established in various studies on rats and mice in ICMR, Lucknow.

64. Pomegranate (Anar)

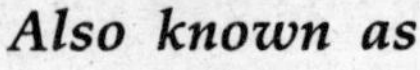

Also known as

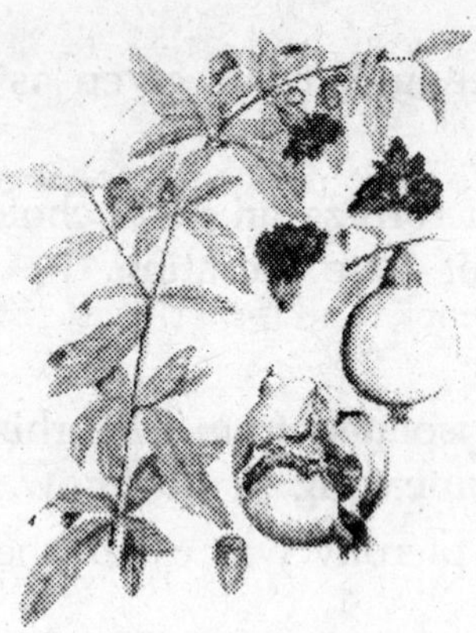

Latin : Punica granatum
English : Pomegranate
Sanskrit : Dadimah
Hindi : Anar
Marathi : Dalimba
Tamil : Madalai
Telugu : Danimma
Malayalam : Talimatalam, Urumampalam
Kannada : Dalimbe

How it looks—It is a large, woody undershrub, with shiny leaves and bright red or sometimes yellow flowers. The fruits are rounded with a tough, woody rind and the inside separated by membranous walls containing numerous red seeds.

What we use—Roots, bark, flowers, fruits, seeds.

What it does—*Root, stem, bark*—astringent, cooling, anthelmintic (especially good against tapeworm)

Flowers—styptic and antiemetic.

Fruits—aphrodisiac, laxative, diuretic

Seeds—diuretic, cardiotonic, anti-emetic

How we use it—

In **bleeding piles**—Take a tsp of the powder of the dry rind of pomegranate with buttermilk to arrest the bleeding.

In **blood in motions and diarrhoea**—A decoction of equal parts of Kutaja bark and pomegranate rind powder is taken with a tsp of honey.

In **distaste**—Saunph and pomegranate seeds should be pasted and held in the mouth to clear the unpleasant taste.

In **tastelessness**—The juice of pomegranate, rock salt and honey should be held in the mouth for a few minutes and then swallowed.

In **bleeding from the mouth**—The powder of the rind of pomegranate fruit should be licked with sugar and honey.

To **prevent abortion**—In threat of abortion during the 5th month of pregnancy, the powder of the leaves of pomegranate and sandal powder should be taken frequently with yoghurt and honey.

To maintain firmness of breasts—An oil is prepared with the paste of the fruit and sesame oil and applied on the breasts regularly to help maintain their firmness.

In **indigestion**—Mix the juice of pomegranate with a tsp of honey and drink to cure conditions of indigestion especially when accompanied by giddiness.

In **nasal bleeding**—Pound the buds with water and instill a few drops in the nose to arrest bleeding.

In **anal itching**—Roast the rind of the fruit until it turns black and powder it. Mix this charred powder in some oil and apply over the anus.

In **tapeworm infection**—Make a decoction of the stem bark and drink. Punicine, the alkaloid in the stem bark is very effective against tapeworms.

To **increase memory**—Dry the flower buds of pomegranate and powder them. Roll the powder into small pills and take a pill thrice a day to enhance memory power.

65. Radish (Muli)

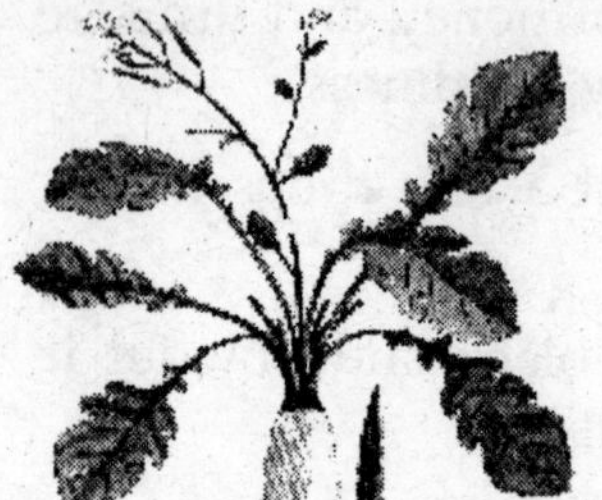

Also known as

Latin	:	**Raphanus sativus**
English	:	**Radish**
Sanskrit	:	**Mulaka**
Hindi	:	**Muli**
Marathi	:	**Mula**
Tamil	:	**Mullanki**
Telugu	:	**Mullangi**
Malayalam	:	**Mullanki**
Kannada	:	**Mulangi**

How it looks—It is an annual or biennial herb with a short condensed stem and a white or brightly coloured tap root. The leaves are long and roughly toothed, the flowers are white and scented and the fruits are erect pods with many seeds.

What we use—Roots, leaves, seeds.

What it does—*Root*—thermogenic, digestive, laxative, anti-inflammatory, antibacterial.
Seeds—expectorant, diuretic, emmenagogue, laxative.

How we use it—

In **jaundice**—White radish juice is given with a tsp of honey twice a day to control the infection.

In **piles**—White radish grated and mixed with a tsp each of honey and ghee every day is a surefire remedy for piles.

Even externally, white radish is ground to a paste in milk and applied over the inflamed masses to relieve pain and swelling.

In **white spots on nails**—Introducing both red and white radishes into regular diet will improve vitamin content and make these white spots disappear in no time.

To **prevent cold**—Regular intake of white radish juice with a tsp of honey is effective in keeping colds at bay.

In **spleen trouble**—Cut root and place ammonium chloride on it. Keep it open for overnight and take in the morning. Repeat for 15 days.

In **urine trouble**—Take radish as a salad with meals. It will help reduce urinary trouble.

66. Saffron (Kesar)

Also known as

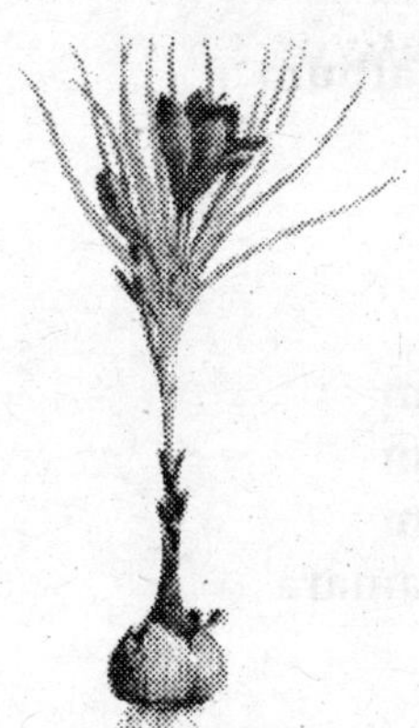

Latin	:	**Crocus sativus**
English	:	**Saffron**
Sanskrit	:	**Kunkumam, Kesaram**
Hindi	:	**Saphran, Kesar**
Marathi	:	**Kesar/Kumkum**
Tamil	:	**Kunkumappu**
Telugu	:	**Kunkumapuvvu**
Malayalam	:	**Kunkumapppuvu**
Kannada	:	**Kunkumakesari**

How it looks—It is a small, bulbous, perennial herb cultivated chiefly in Jammu and Kashmir, with close narrow leaf sheaths. The flowers are blue and scented with orange trifid stigmas having a characteristic aroma.

What we use—Dried stigmas.

The styles and stigmas which are dried are called saffron.

What it does—Stimulant, tonic, stomachic, aphrodisiac, antispasmodic, emmenogogue, diuretic, laxative, galactogogue.

How we use it—

In **cold**—Saffron mixed in milk and applied over the forehead quickly relieves cold. Breastmilk is ideal in this condition.

In **patchy baldness**—Saffron mixed in liquorice and milk makes an effective topical application to induce hair growth in alopecia.

In **delayed puberty**—In underdeveloped girls, saffron has an overall stimulating effect. A pinch of saffron crushed in a tablespoon of milk is useful to stimulate hormones and bring about the desired effect.

In **pregnancy**—Probably the most renowned use of saffron is its ability to promote complexion. It is widely used all over India in pregnancy to ensure the birth of a fair baby. A pinch of saffron in milk every day is the recommended dose, but should be discontinued on signs of overheat or spotty bleeding.

To **increase vitality**—In low libido, saffron aids as a sexual stimulant and is consumed in a dose of a pinch in a glass of milk at bedtime.

67. Sandal (Chandan)

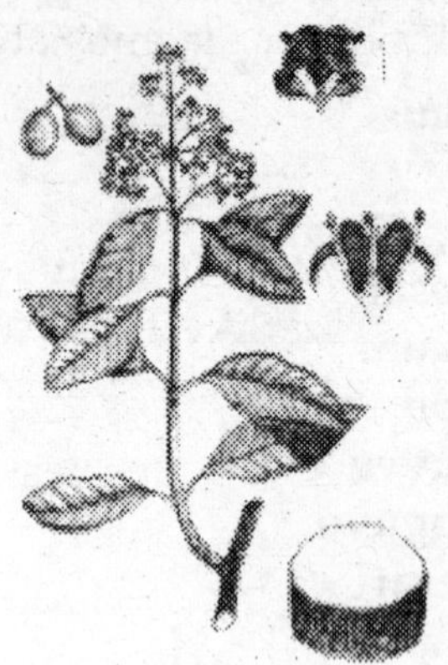

Also known as

Latin	**:**	**Santalum album**
English	**:**	**Sandal**
Sanskrit	**:**	**Candanah**
Hindi	**:**	**Chandan**
Marathi	**:**	**Chandan**
Tamil	**:**	**Chandanam**
Telugu	**:**	**Chandanam**
Malayalam	**:**	**Chandanam**
Kannada	**:**	**Srigandadamara**

"That which delights" is the meaning of the Sanskrit word chandana

RED SANDAL—Pterocarpus santalinus
Santanal 90% in sandal oil.

How it looks—It is a medium sized evergreen tree, with slender drooping branches and yellowish brown heartwood which is highly scented.

What we use—Heartwood

What it does—It is deodorant, demulcent, cosmetic and coolant.

How we use it—

In **menorrhagia, white vaginal discharge, spermatorrhoea, difficulty in urination, chronic thirst**—Take the decoction of the heartwood of sandal to cool the system and arrest excessive fluid discharges.

In **allergic rashes, burning sensation, headaches, jaundice, hyperacidity, discolourations, chronic cough.**—As a soothing and cooling application sandal enjoys a special place especially in tropical countries such as ours.It is a very well known cosmetic as it tones and clears the skin.

In **hiccups**—Take the decoction of sandal internally and instill a few drops in the nostrils.

In **eye disorders**—Paste chandan with a few drops of breastmilk and instill the same in the eyes to reduce inflammations and tone the eyes.

WHITE SANDAL

How it looks—It is a medium sized evergreen tree with slender drooping branches and dark grey to brownish black bark which have vertical cracks. The flowers are brownish purple or violet in colour and the fruits are rounded purplish-black drupes with hard seeds. The heart wood is light yellowish brown when fresh, and turns dark reddish brown on exposure, having a characteristic deep fragrance.

What we use—Heartwood

What it does—Aromatic, deodorant, disinfectant, refrigerant, cardiotonic, intellect promoting, diuretic, diaphoretic, expectorant, aphrodisiac, haemostatic, antipyretic, restorative and tonic.

How we use it—

In **prickly heat**—To steer clear of prickly heat and to keep the body cool in summer, apply a paste of sandal over the body especially in hot, sweaty areas like forehead, armpits, groins, back etc. It prevents excessive sweating by contracting the pores.

In **headaches**—Apply a thin layer of sandal paste and camphor over the temples to relieve throbbing pain.

In **fevers**—A paste of pachakarpooram or edible camphor and sandal is applied over the body to reduce temperature.

In **dysuria**—Make a decoction of sandal powder and drink a glass twice a day to facilitate urination and soothe accompanying burning sensation and pain.

In **blood accompanying urine**—A combination of sandal and madder (manjith) is good in reddish urination.

In **spermatorrhoea**—Sandal powder should be mixed with a decoction of Arjuna bark and taken everyday to prevent spermatorrhoea.

In **menorrhagea and white discharge**—A tsp of sandal powder is mixed in a glass of milk with ghee, honey and sugar and taken twice a day to correct heavy menstrual flow.

In **diarrhoea and dysentery**—Mix a tsp of sandal powder in rice wash along with honey and sugar to arrest loose motions and accompanying bleeding.

In all **allergic rashes and discolourations**—The sandal paste should be applied regularly to discolourations while a single application may suffice to soothe a rash or itching eruptions.

In **hiccups**—Mix a pinch of sandal in breastmilk and instill a few drops in the nose to control hiccups.

In **jaundice and hyperacidity**—The decoction of sandal wood should be taken from time to time as a coolant and to flush out toxins.

Modern Studies

1. The aqueous extract of the bark exhibited antibacterial activity against Staphylococcus aureus and Escherichia coli.
2. Sandal powder, as a Siddha drug was clinically tried on non-insulin dependent diabetes mellitus patients in New Delhi. A significant fall in blood sugar levels was observed after 45 days of treatment.

68. Sarsaparilla (Anantamul)

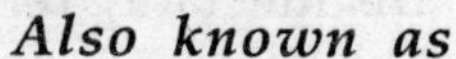

Also known as

Latin	:	**Hemidesmus indicus**
English	:	**Sarsaparilla**
Sanskrit	:	**Anantamulah, Sariba**
Hindi	:	**Anantamul**
Marathi	:	**Upalasari**
Tamil	:	**Nannari**
Telugu	:	**Sugandhipala**
Malayalam	:	**Nannari**
Kannada	:	**Namadaballi**

How it looks—It is a slender, perennial, turning, wiry shrub with a woody root stock and numerous slender stems having thickened nodes. The leaves are long and lance shaped, white striped above and silvery white below. The flowers are greenish purple and fruits are slender cylindrical and tapering.

The tuberous root is dark-brown, silvery white inside with twisted, fissured bark. It has a strong, pleasant smell and taste.

What we use—Roots, leaves, stem

What it does—Roots—aromatic, refrigerant, aphrodisiac, carminative, appetiser, demulcent, febrifuge, expectorant, tonic.

How we use it—

In **piles**—Make the following preparation for daily use in piles. Ferment milk to curds in a mud vessel along with the root of sarsaparilla put in it. Use this curd to prepare buttermilk for use in daily diet to obtain relief from piles.

In **wounds**—Wash wounds with a decoction of sarsaparilla leaves and roots to hasten recovery.

In **body heat and burning sensation**—Boil ghee with sarsaparilla roots and take a tsp of this ghee in milk every day on empty stomach.

A decoction of the root will also serve the purpose.

In **breathlessness or asthma**—Use the same sarsaparilla- cooked ghee in hot milk to reduce respiratory spasms and allergy.

In **corneal ulcers/eye inflammations**—Wash eyes with a mixture of the decoction of Sarsaparilla roots and some honey for its astringent action.

In **paralysis, joint pains and nervous disorders**—Mix the powder of sarsaparilla root and vasaka leaves in some milk and drink everyday. This lubricates joints, enables free movements and is strengthening to the nerves.

In **diarrhoea and dysentery**—Mix a tsp of the root powder in a glass of buttermilk and drink it from time to time to arrest loose motions.

In **skin discolourations**—Make a pack of the root powder and milk and apply to the face regularly for a blemish – free complexion.

69. Serpentina (Candrabhaga)

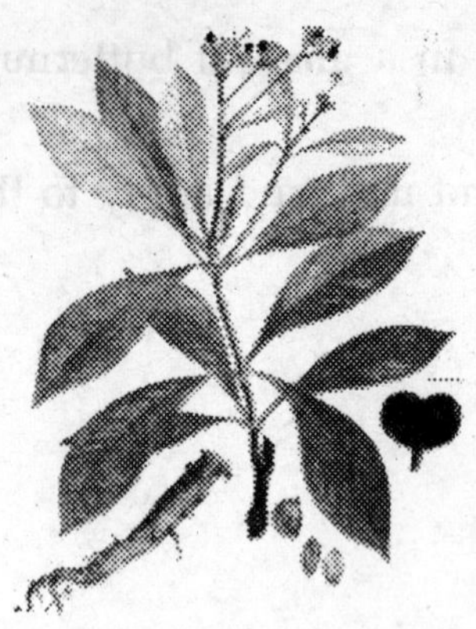

Also known as

Latin	:	**Rauvolfia serpentina**
English	:	**Serpentina root**
Sanskrit	:	**Sarpagandha**
Hindi	:	**Candrabhaga**
Marathi	:	**Hadaki/Adakai**
Tamil	:	**Sarpagandha**
Telugu	:	**Patalagandha**
Malayalam	:	**Amalpori**
Kannada	:	**Sutranabhi**

How it looks—It is a small erect shrub with wholly, bright green leaves, white flowers often tinged with violet and purplish black fruits (when ripe). The dry roots are very hard and yield a yellowish paste upon rubbing with water.

What we use—Roots

What it does—*Roots*—laxative, anthelmintic

> **Caution:** Serpentina can cause constipation when taken over a long periods and so it is recommended to take 1 tsp of triphala with warm water at bedtime during its use.

How we use it—

In **high blood pressure**—Reserpine present in sarpagandha has recently been introduced as an antihypertensive to the modern system of medicine. Take half a tsp of the powdered root twice a day to control hypertension.

In **fever with fits and hysteria**—Take a pinch of the root powder in warm milk thrice a day until symptoms completely disappear.

In **insanity**—Owing to its sedative effects, sarpagandha enjoys a prominent place in the treatment of schizophrenia, especially when associated with violent behaviour and hypertension. Give a pinch of the root powder with cows milk and sugar candy twice a day. Blood pressure should be monitored throughout the treatment. It is best avoided in depressed and hypotensive patients.

In **sleeplessness**—Again as a well-known sedative, very minute doses of serpentina–about half a gram-can be taken along with some buffalo's milk at bedtime. It induces sound sleep–especially in those suffering from phlegm afflicting the chest and painful joints.

In **itching skin**—Sarpagandha taken in doses of a pinch twice a day with decoction of kutja or plain water soothes the urge to scratch.

70. Shoe Flower (Jasum)

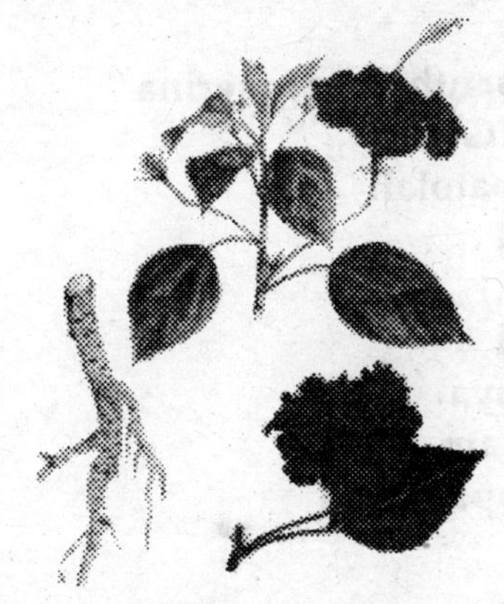

Also known as

Latin	:	**Hibiscus rosa sinensis**
English	:	**Shoe Flower**
Sanskrit	:	**Japa**
Hindi	:	**Jasum**
Marathi	:	**Jaswanda**
Tamil	:	**Chemparutti**
Telugu	:	**Mandaram**
Malayalam	:	**Tavilamma**
Kannada	:	**Sanadika**

How it looks—It is an evergreen woody shrub with pale grey or whitish bark. The leaves are bright green and the flowers are single, bright red and showy.

What we use—Roots, leaves, flowers.

What it does—*Roots*—febrifuge demulcent

Leaves—refrigerant, emollient, depurative

Flowers—astringent, emollient, demulcent, aphrodisiac, emmenagogue, haemostatic, brain tonic, cardiotonic.

How we use it—

In **jaundice**—Hibiscus flowers, neem leaves, keezhanelli leaves and white radish are made into a decoction (concentrated to ½ the volume) to relieve even acute cases of jaundice.

In **inflamed skin**—For allergic or infective rashes hibiscus leaf juice/extract in paste acts as an effective topical wash.

In **urticaria**—Grind red hibiscus flowers in water and apply over the swellings.

In Hair care—

1. Hibiscus leaf juice is good to wash hair with and is a popular ingredient of many hair care preparations.
   - Removes excess oil
   - Keeps lice at bay
   - Nourishes hair
2. Red hibiscus flowers partially dried and boiled in coconut oil make an excellent hair dye.

As a **cardiac tonic**—A decoction of the flowers mixed in milk and sugar makes for an effective heart tonic, when taken on empty stomach.

71. Snake Gourd (Paraval)

Also known as

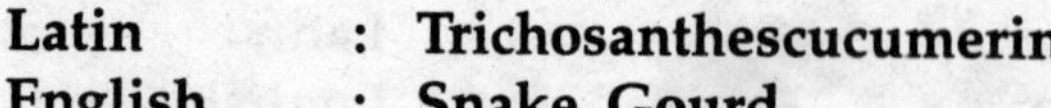

Latin	:	**Trichosanthescucumerina**
English	:	**Snake Gourd**
Sanskrit	:	**Svadupatolah**
Hindi	:	**Paraval**
Marathi	:	**Palasa**
Tamil	:	**Putaval**
Telugu	:	**Potlakaya**
Malayalam	:	**Patavalam**
Kannada	:	**Bettadapadavala**

How it looks—It is an annual slender – stemmed climber with large heart-shaped leaves and white flowers. The fruits are green and white striped, changing to orange when ripe and twisted many times. Seeds are many in the fleshy pulp and are hard and yellowish brown.

What we use—Whole plant

What it does—It is cooling, anthelmentic, purgative, vermifuge, febrifuge, digestive, carminative and tonic.

How we use it—

In **vomiting**—Take the juice of the snake gourd with a tsp of honey to mitigate vomiting sensation.

In **burning urination**—Soak the whole plant in water overnight after cutting it into pieces and drink this water in the morning. This is excellent in relieving urethral inflammation and in such conditions as gonorrhoea.

In **fever**—It is the most recommended diet during fever owing to its cooling, digestive and febrifuge properties.
Make a decoction of equal quantities of snake gourd and fresh coriander leaves and drink an ounce or two of this mixture three times a day to reduce high temperature.

In **fungal infections**—Make a paste of snake ground and gramflour and apply it to the infected skin. Wait for the application to dry and wash off with warm water. Pat dry. A few days of this treatment is usually sufficient for cure.

72. Sugarcane (Ganna)

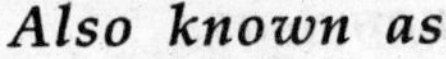

Also known as

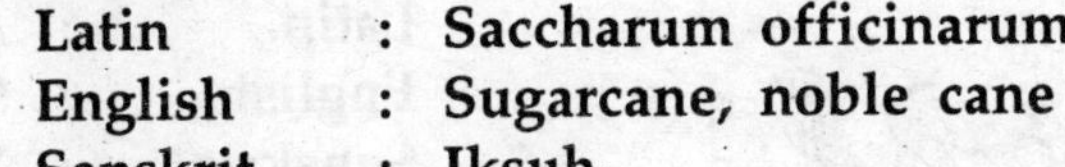

Latin	:	Saccharum officinarum
English	:	Sugarcane, noble cane
Sanskrit	:	Iksuh
Hindi	:	Ganna
Marathi	:	Usa
Tamil	:	Pundaram
Telugu	:	Cheruku
Malayalam	:	Karinpu
Kannada	:	Kabbu

How it looks—It is a graceful, tall perennial grass with stems of varying thickness and colour - ranging from light to dark green.

What we use—Roots, stems

What it does—*Stem*—Sweet, cooling, laxative, diuretic, aphrodisiac, cardiotonic, galactogogue

Roots—cooling, diuretic

How we use it—

In **jaundice**—Sugarcane juice is given in plenty to one suffering from jaundice, to promote urination and flush out toxins. You could combine it with lime juice to hasten recovery.

In **excessive bleeding from any orifice**—Cane juice is considered haematinic and thereby arrests bleeding when consumed from time to time.

In **anaemia**—Supplement a nutritious diet with cane juice for the same reason as above, to improve the blood picture in anaemia.

In **erysipelas**—Slightly heat the juice and sprinkle it on the affected skin to soothe eruptions and hasten healing.

In **dysuria**—The juice of cane being the best among diuretics, it is ideal to consume it thrice a day in any urinary problems including calculi, burning sensation in urine and pain during urination.

To promote flow of breastmilk—Being an effective galactogogue it clears the ducts of the mammary gland and promotes secretion of milk.

Modern Study

Sugarcane was clinically tested and found to be highly effective in the treatment of urinary tract infections.

73. Sweet Flag (Gorbach)

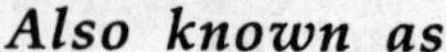

Also known as

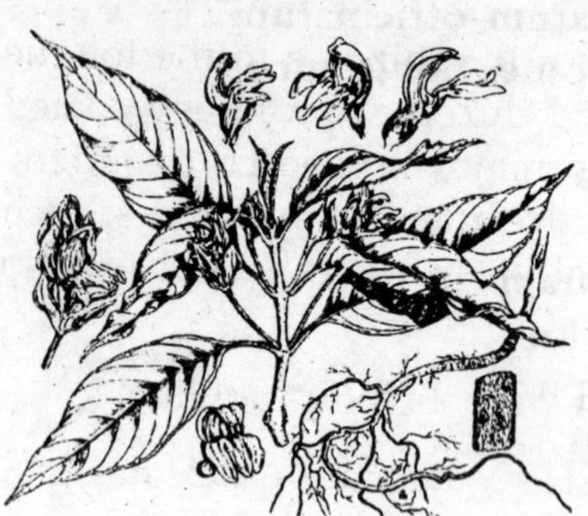

Latin	:	Acorus calamus
English	:	Sweet Flag
Sanskrit	:	Vacha, Ugragandha
Hindi	:	Bach, Gorbach
Marathi	:	Vekhanda
Tamil	:	Vasampu
Telugu	:	Vasa
Malayalam	:	Vayampu
Kannada	:	Baji

"Bestows clear voice"RT is the meaning of the Sanskrit word vacha.

How it looks—It is a semi-aquatic rhizomatous herb, with much-branched creeping rhizomes. The rhizome is cylindrical, light brown externally and spongy white within. The leaves are bright green, arising from the base ,thick in the middle with wavy margins. The flowers are light brown without stalks and the fruits are oblong berries.

What we use—*Rhizomes*

What it does—It is thermogenic, aromatic, intellect promoting, emetic, laxative, carminative, anthelmentic, emmenagogue, diuretic, expectorant, antispasmodic, aphrodisiac, anticonvulsant, anti-inflammatory and anti-pyretic.

How we use it—

In **abdominal pain**—Paste bach, nutmeg and harad and take half a tsp of this as a digestive and antispasmodic. This can also be given to in dysmenorrhoea to relieve pain and promote flow of blood.

In **worm infestation**—Especially in infants when it is difficult to choose a safe medicine, a pinch of bach powder mixed in honey acts as a wonderful dewormant and may be used every month.

In **diarrhoea and dysentery**—The high content of essential oils and tannins make it a useful medicine .Paste the bach with buttermilk and drink it down to arrest loose motions and relieve griping pains accompanying.

In **colds**—In small doses, bach acts as expectorant by diluting phlegm and easing it out. For this vacha should be ground with honey and half a tea spoonful licked down. You could also inhale the vapours of bach ground and added to boiling water.

In **cough**—Even in whooping cough, the following recipe is useful. Roast the rhizome, and powder it and give a pinch of the powder with honey in children suffering from whooping cough, to prevent severe bouts.

In **oral ulcers and coating of tongue**—Rub a small piece of the rhizome in the tongue and cheeks to soothe oral ulcers. The dried and powdered rhizome and honey coated on the tongue ,inside of cheeks and palate is excellent in removing speech disorders. This practice is followed in new born children to improve intellect and for speech clarity, and also in people affected by paralysis and facial palsy where speech is also disturbed.

In **inflammation**—honey and ghee should be mixed in bach before applying.

In **wounds**—The powder is used for dusting on wounds to facilitate quick healing.

In **swellings**—Paste mustard and bach in water and apply on inflammatory swellings.

74. Tamarind (Imli)

Also known as

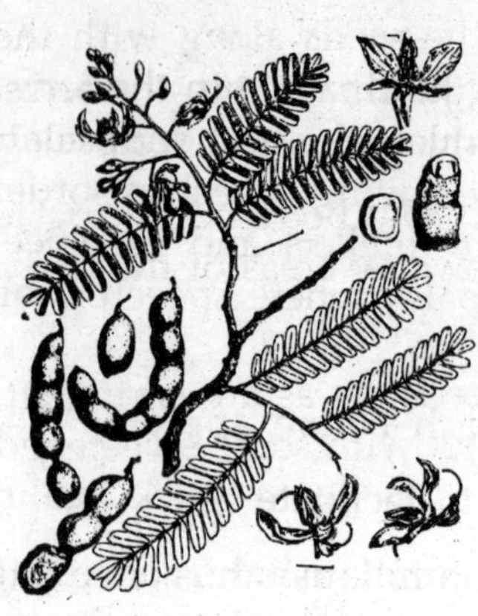

Latin	:	**Tamarindus indicus**
English	:	**Tamarind tree**
Sanskrit	:	**Cinca, Tintrini**
Hindi	:	**Imli**
Marathi	:	**Chincha**
Tamil	:	**Puli Amilam**
Telugu	:	**Chintapandu**
Malayalam	:	**Puli, Kolpuli**
Kannada	:	**Huli, Amli**

How it looks—It is a large evergreen tree with tiny leaflets, yellow flowers, and pod fruits.

What we use—Roots, leaves, fruits, seeds.

What it does—*Root bark*—astringent, emmenagogue, constipating

Leaves—astringent, anthelmintic, anti-inflammatory, antifungal, diuretic.

Fruits—refrigerant, digestive, carminative, laxative, antiseptic

How we use it—

In **infections and fevers**—Drink the juice of the leaves with some turmeric powder and cold water everyday to cleanse the system of infections and micro-organisms.

In **fractures**—The fruit of tamarind is pasted with sesame oil and applied as a warm poultice over the fractured area.

In **swelling and hernias**—Paste the leaves of tamarind and apply on swellings twice a day to bring them down.

Ripe fruit is specific for **intoxication** from liquors or dhatura.

In **earaches**—A few drops of the fruit juice of tamarind should be instilled in the ear after slightly warming to foment and soothe the ear.

In **excessive white discharge**—Soak some tamarind seeds in a glass of water overnight. Paste the soaked seeds in some milk the next morning and drink it. This treatment, when followed for a few weeks stops white discharge completely.

In **itching**—In any condition of itching, apply the juice of the leaves on the affected skin to allay the irritation.

In **anal fistula**—Apply a paste of the seeds of tamarind everyday in case of fistula-in-ano

In **rectal prolapse**—Steam the seeds of tamarind and paste the seeds along with the flowers to apply on the prolapsed rectum. Push the projecting part back into the anus. Repeat this procedure everyday for a few weeks to prevent mucoceles and rectoceles.

In **offensive body odour**—To prevent excessive sweating and foul body odour, paste the ripe fruits of tamarind with its flowers and apply on the sweaty areas of the body. This helps close the pores and prevents body odour.

In **diarrhoea**—Though the fruit of tamarind is laxating, the seeds act as an astringent. Powder 5-6 tamarind seeds with a tsp of cumin seeds and drink with some sweetened water to arrest loose motions.

In **burns**—Burn the leaves of tamarind in a closed pot. Finely sieve the ash thus obtained and mix with sesame oil and apply over the burnt part for quick healing.

In **sprains**—Apply a thick paste of tamarind with lots of salt on the sprained area to prevent swelling and pain.

75. Tea (Chay)

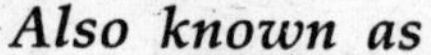

Also known as

Latin	:	**Camellia thea**
English	:	**Tea Plant**
Sanskrit	:	**Syamaparni, caha**
Hindi	:	**Chay**
Marathi	:	**Chaha**
Tamil	:	**Teyilai**
Telugu	:	**Teyaku**
Malayalam	:	**Teyila**
Kannada	:	**Teyaku**

How it looks—It is an evergreen shrub or tree, about 9-15m in height with leathery, oily leaves and white fragrant flowers. The fruits are 3 cornered and 3 seeded.

What we use—Leaves

What it does—It is digestive, carminative, diuretic and a nervine tonic

How we use it—

> **How to prepare a healthy tea infusion**—Contrary to general prevalence, tea leaves should never be boiled in water. Put some tea leaves in a kettle and pour hot water into it. After a few minutes, filter this water and add milk and sugar according to preference before drinking.

Origin of Tea—Mythology from China

One day, the Buddha was trying to focus his thoughts to meditate when sleep kept overwhelming him. After repeated efforts in vain, the Buddha, stood up decisively, cut off both lids from his eyes and flung them on the ground. Lo! A sapling sprung up from the very place. Intrigued, he plucked a few leaves from the young plant and ate them. To his surprise, he felt invigorated immediately and could easily concentrate on his objective. This young sapling came to be known, later, as tea, which is why the Chinese hold tea to be a divine drink and even allot a special room in the house for tea drinking [Source : Camphor]

How we use it—

In **fatigue and listlessness**—Possibly the most popular use of tea is to banish sleep and infuse freshness in the mind and activity of the drinker. The method of preparation is given in the box.

In heart diseases—Drinking an infusion of tea leaves everyday is highly beneficial to the heart and has recently been medically proved to be a cardiac tonic.

In **cold and throat irritation**—Drinking ginger tea is quite prevalent in India at the first sign of cold or sore throat. Add a few crushed pieces of fresh ginger to water boiling for tea, and then make the tea.

In **dysentery accompanied by pain**—The decoction of tea with a tsp of ghee works wonderfully to heal inflammation of intestines in case of blood and mucous in stool.

In **tonsilitis**—A gargle of tannin-rich tea is effective in healing sore throat and tonsillitis. This treatment is especially followed in hilly regions.

In **fevers**—Caffeine in tea acts as a diuretic and brings down temperature.

In **eye inflammation**—A brew of tea leaves, can be used as an eye wash, after filtration, and brings down irritation and swelling quickly.

In **eczema**—Wash the lesions twice a day with a solution of tea and rock salt. This can be followed by applying a paste of fenugreek seeds and Rakta chandan (red variety of sandal wood)

To dye hair—Tea extract serves as a good hair dye and rinsing hair with concentrated tea decoction, at least twice a week, ensures that grey hair turns brown or black.

Tea is rich source of—

1. Beta-carotene, an anti-oxidant.
2. Vitamin B_1, Vitamin B_2 and Vitamin B_6.
3. Nicotinic acid and pantothemic acid.
4. Vitamin C, an anti-oxidant.
5. Folic acid.
6. Maganese and
7. Potassium.

76. Tinospora/Giloy

Also known as

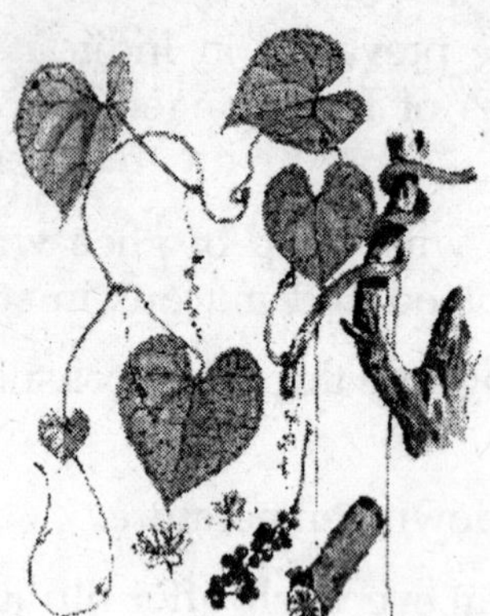

Latin	**:**	**Tinospora cordifolia**
English	**:**	**Tinospora**
Sanskrit	**:**	**Amrta, Guduci**
Hindi	**:**	**Giloy**
Marathi	**:**	**Gulavela**
Tamil	**:**	**Amrutavalli**
Telugu	**:**	**Tippa tiga**
Malayalam	**:**	**Cittamrtu**
Kannada	**:**	**Amrtaballi**

How it looks—It is a large, extensively spreading twiner with a woody succulent stem and papery bark. The leaves are typically heart- shaped and the flowers are yellow arising from the nodes. The fruits are drupes and turn red when ripe. The surface of the stems appears warty and is fissured longitudinally.

What we use—Stem

What it does—It has a wide range of properties such as bitter, astringent, sweet, thermogenic, anodyne, anthelmentic, alterant antispasmodic, anti-inflammatory, antipyretic, anti-emetic, digestive, carminative, appetiser, haematinic, expectorant, aphrodisiac, galacto purifier and tonic.

How we use it—

In **fevers**—It is commonly used in fevers of any origin. The fresh stem is more effective than the dry one. The decoction of the fresh stem should be taken in doses of an ounce thrice a day in fevers. You could also squeeze the juice of the stem and drink it diluted twice a day.

It is also useful in debility caused by repeated attacks of fever.

In **rheumatism**—A decoction made of a tsp each of tinospora and dry ginger is very useful in rheumatic pain. Drink an ounce before meals twice a day.

In **all skin disorders**—Being alterative, tinospora is highly useful in all skin disorders including early stages of leprosy. Again the fresh juice expressed from the stem, or its decoction is used.

In **liver disorders**—As a liver tonic, a vegetable curry made of the leaves and stems of tinospora are included in diet in conditions such as jaundice.

In **piles**—The same vegetable curry mentioned above serves as a digestive and promotes bowel movement and is therefore highly recommended in piles.

As **an aphrodisiac**—The juice of tinospora is also useful as a general tonic and aphrodisiac.

In **systemic disorders**—Being nutritive and alterative, it can be used with great benefits in consumption, hormonal imbalance, diabetes and other wasting diseases.

Modern Study

Improvement in neutrophil function was noticed after administering tinospora to mice in experimental studies in **Cancer Research institute,** Bombay.

77. Turmeric (Haldi)

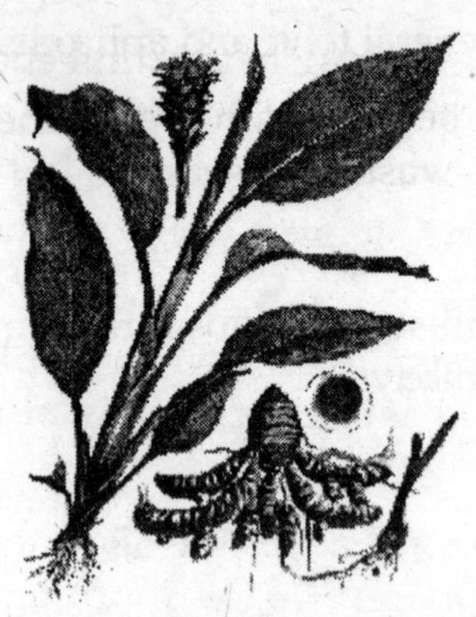

Also known as

Latin	:	**Curcuma longa**
English	:	**Turmeric**
Sanskrit	:	**Haridra**
Hindi	:	**Haldi**
Marathi	:	**Halada**
Tamil	:	**Mancal**
Telugu	:	**Pasupu**
Malayalam	:	**Mannal**
Kannada	:	**Arisina**

How it looks—It is a small perennial herb, with a short stem and a tuft of erect, pointing leaves. The rhizome is orange cylindrical and branched.

What we use—Rhizome - both fresh and dry

What it does—It is thermogenic, anti-inflamnatory antiseptic, anthelmintic, appetizer, diuretic, laxative, expectorant and carminative

How we use it—

In **diabetes**—One tsp of turmeric powder along with some gooseberry juice taken everyday is quite effective in keeping blood glucose levels under control.

In **fevers**—A decoction of a tsp of turmeric powder, some ginger pieces and half a tsp of black pepper in about 8 ounces of water should be taken thrice a day to bring down fever.

In **colds**—Add turmeric powder with some pepper and jaggery to a glass of hot milk and take thrice a day to relieve congestion and cure colds. Alternately you could add a tsp of turmeric and a quarter tsp of ajwoin to a cup of boiling water and take it after cooling with some honey.

In cough and throat irritation—Half a tsp of pure turmeric powder in an ounce of warm milk is a common household drink for coughs. Make a concentrated solution of turmeric with a pinch of rock salt and coat this on the inside of the inflamed throat for quick healing.

In **diarrhoea and dysentery**—A pinch of turmeric and rock salt is to be added to dilute buttermilk and consumed to set right an upset stomach. Turmeric, being a gastric stimulant, as well as, a blood enricher is ideally suited for this condition.

In **wounds**—A most popular remedy to arrest bleeding in fresh wounds is to plug the site with some turmeric powder. Quick lime can also be added to turmeric to hasten the effect.

In **fungal infections/scabies**—A paste of turmeric is applied especially in infections affecting the crevices of the fingers and toes. The known antibacterial, antifungal and antiviral properties of turmeric make it the first and best choice in such conditions.

In urticaria, taking a fresh piece of turmeric rhizome on empty stomach every morning goes a long way in curing the eruptions.

As a **depilatory**—Turmeric is best known for its cosmetic value and when applied as an ubtan regularly, not only keeps skin free of acne and infections, but is also a safe and natural hair - remover.

In **blackheads**—Turmeric and mustard seeds are pasted and touched on the blackheads and left on overnight. The face is washed clear with gramflour in the morning.

In **worm infestations**—A paste of turmeric and curry leaves is rolled into a ball and swallowed twice a day to get rid of intestinal worms.

In **urinary calculi**—Turmeric powder with a little jaggery should be consumed with "kanji" (rice gruel) twice a day.

In **mumps**—A paste of neem leaves and turmeric is a popular external application on the swollen glands.

In **bronchitis**—Take one tsp turmeric powder with warm water 3 times a day.

In **piles**—Take one teaspoonful turmeric powder with water in the morning and evening.

In **cosmetic cream**—Mix equal amount of turmeric powder and gram flour in curd. Make a paste. Apply over the face to get relief from acne and black spots.

Modern Studies

1. The ethereal extract of turmeric inhibited platelet aggression in an experimental study thereby proving its anti-inflammatory property.
2. Turmeric was established as an effective dietary supplement in clinical trials on non-insulin dependant diabetics.
3. It has been shown in the National Institute of Nutrition, Hyderabad that curcumin extracted from turmeric exhibited anti-cancer activities.

78. Winter Cherry (Ashwagandha)

Also known as

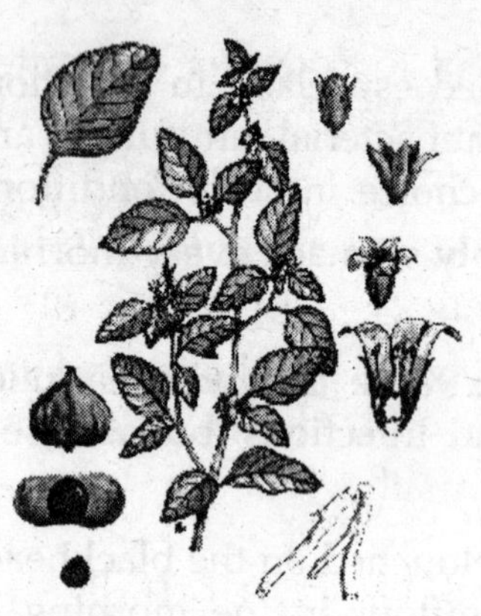

Latin	:	**Withania somnifera**
English	:	**Winter cherry**
Sanskrit	:	**Ashwagandha**
Hindi	:	**Ashwagandha**
Marathi	:	**Askandha/Bhuikohala**
Tamil	:	**Amukkira**
Telugu	:	**Vajigandha, Pennerugadda**
Malayalam	:	**Amukkuram**
Kannada	:	**Veramaddinagaddi**

Introduction—It is popularly known as Indian ginseng. Ashwagandha has an ancient history and acquired much folklore praise on its actions and uses. It is cultivated in China and Korea etc.,

How it looks—It is an erect branching undershrub with ovate leaves and greenish/yellow flowers. The fruits are orange coloured when ripe and are rounded berries. The fleshy roots are cylindrical, with a brownish white surface and white inside.

What we use—Roots, leaves

What it does—Roots-astringent, somniferous, stimulant, aphrodisiac, diuretic, thermogenic, tonic.

How we use it—

It is a widely accepted herb with a global market as "Indian ginseng". It is found in dry wastelands and is also cultivated extensively in Rajasthan and Madhya Pradesh for its much-in-demand tuberous roots. Its wide range of medicinal use is reflected in the Telugu proverb, " Peru leni vyadhiki pennerugadda"or "for a´nameless disease ashwagandha is the medicine."

In **impotence and low sperm count**—Probably the most publicised use of Ashwagandha is its effect on the male reproductive system. Take a tsp of the root powder with warm milk everyday for sexual vitality and to improve the sperm count.

In **low body weight and weakness**—Ashwagandha can be prepared as a lehyam (confectionery) with sugar candy crystals, ghee and honey. A tsp of this lehyam should be taken everyday with warm milk for tissue building and to enhance general strength.

As a **nervine tonic**—The same lehya preparation can be taken in doses of a tsp twice a day for nervine disorders such as hysteria, epilepsy, and even parkinsonism.

In **leucoderma**—It is a good supportive drug for treatment of leucoderma or white patches. Ashwagandharishta available in the market should be taken in doses of 20ml twice a day after food.

In **painful joints and boils**—Heat the leaves of Ashwagandha and apply on painful joints while still warm to relieve ache.

In **poisoning**—Ashwagandha is given as an antidote for aconite poisoning and to eliminate toxins accumulated in the system due to syphilis or other chronic ailments.

As a special use it raises the lowered blood pressure to normal level.

Modern Studies

All the alkaloids and steroidal lactones present in the crude drug have been investigated for different biological activities.

1. Free radical scavenging activity of Ashwagandha root powder was found in 15 days of experimental studies on rats. This was suggested to be responsible for its pharmacological effects.
2. Hepato protective and nephro protective (liver and kidney protective) roles of Ashwagandha were proved in metal- induced toxicity in experimental studies on mice in Indore.
3. Ashwagandha tablets improved the physical and mental health of pre-school children in clinical trials in Chennai.

79. Wood Apple (Kaith)

Also known as

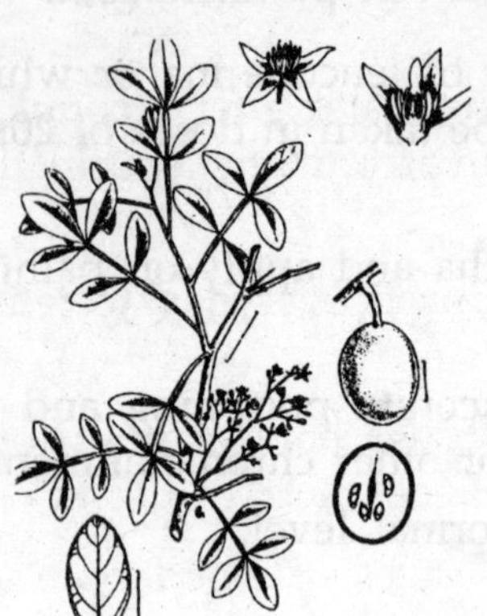

Latin	:	**Feronia elephantum**
English	:	**Elephant Apple, wood Apple**
Sanskrit	:	**Kapithah**
Hindi	:	**Kaith**
Marathi	:	**Kavatha**
Tamil	:	**Vilankaymaram**
Telugu	:	**Velagapandu**
Malayalam	:	**Vilarmaram**
Kannada	:	**Bela**

How it looks—

It is a moderately sized to large woody tree armed with strong straight spines at the axils and a dense crown of dark foliage. The leaves are gland- dotted and the flowers are fragrant, small and dull red in terminal panicles. The fruits are rounded, woody, rough and grey with oblong seeds embedded in the pulp.

"Feronia gum" is obtained from the trunk and branches after the rainy season which is transparent and reddish-brown in colour.

What we use— *Bark*—aromatic, cooling

Leaves—aromatic, astringent, carminative, constipating, antiemetic, expectorant and cardio tonic

Unripe—sour, aromatic, astringent ,constipating

Ripe—sweet, sour, refrigerant, aromatic, anodyne, constipating, aphrodisiac, cardiotonic, antiscorbutic, expectorant, stomachic

How we use it—

In **bronchitis and hiccough**—Make a decoction of the leaves and drink an ounce twice a day with honey to expectorate phlegm, clear airways and reduce irritability.

In **heart ailments**—Drink half an ounce of decoction made of the woodapple leaves with milk everyday to tone your heart.

In **diarrhoea and dysentery**—Woodapple is constipating in nature and is used with great benefits in an upset stomach. Soak the fruit in water for an hour and mash the fruit in the same water before drinking. This quickly arrests diarrhoea and restores digestion.

In **bleeding conditions**—The ripe woodapple is a rich source of Vitamin 'C' and can be given as such in bleeding gums or any excessive bleeding condition. It can also be fried in ghee.

In **dysuria**—Soak the ripe woodapple in water and drink the water after a couple of hours with some sugar. This relieves burning sensation and pain accompanying urination. This preparation also quenches long standing thirsts.

In **piles**—Make an infusion of bael and woodapple and drink it everyday to relieve piles.

In **vomiting**—Juice the tender leaves of woodapple, add pepper powder and honey and lick this preparation from time to time to suppress nausea and vomiting.

In **discolourations**—Grind a few coriander seeds with the leaves of woodapple and apply to skin patches to lighten them.

In **tastelessness**—Eat the pulp of a ripe wood apple with honey and saunph seeds to remove distaste and improve taste sensation..

In **white discharge**—Juice the leaves of woodapple and bamboo or powder the dried leaves and take them with honey.

In **hiccough**—Crushing tender leaves of woodapple in the palm and sniffing it up the nostrils arrests hiccough immediately.

4.

Disease-Wise Green Remedies for Common Problems

Aches and Pains

Aches and pains are the symptoms of deeper problems of health. Herbal / Green Remedies can do more than just relieving the pain, many of them repair and rejunuvate the damaged organs / tissues.

S. No.	Complaint	Green Remedies	Actions	Uses/ Dosage	Combination	Cautions	Equivalent Market Preparations
1	2	3	4	5	6	7	8
1.	**ARTHRITIS** (Joint Pains) It is mainly of 2 types. **(1) Osteo-Arthritis (OA)** is pain and swelling of the joints due to wear and tear	1. Guggulu – the resin of Commiphora mukul	Anti – inflammatory pain killer	250mg hand rolled pills. 2 pills twice a day with warm milk.	In OA, Guggulu & Asgandha for internal use and Nirgundi oil for external application	Larger doses may cause heat or bleeding	Yograj guggul
	(2) Rheumatoid Arthritis (RA) is inflamma-tion of many joints	2. Ashwagandha Root powder of Withania somnifera.	Controls vata dosha	5 grams / 1tsp of fine powder well mixed in a cup of milk.	---	---	R'compound tabs

	manifested due to systemic causes. Requires professional treatment under an expert rheumatologist / Ayurvedic Physician. In general rheumatism refers to any muscle pain. This aggravates in the damp weather. **Specific Symptoms:** Stiff and painful joints Cracking sounds in joints Swollen or deformed joints Hot / burning joints (RA)	3.Nirgundi, (sambhal) leaves of Vitex negundo	Anti vata pro hostic	Oil prepared from Nirgundi leaves can be applied on the affected joints.	—	—	Nirgundi Tail Maha narayana tail for gentle massage
		4.Garlic bulb cloves - bulb of Allium sativum	Confirmed anti arthritic analgesic and anti - inflammatory action	It can be used as drink with milk (Lasunadivati)	Garlic clove + milk or Garlic clove + butter	Avoid in ulcer / acidity	Garlic pearls Lasunadi Vati
2.	**SPRAINS & STRAINS** Injuries to joints and stretch of muscles,	Garlic	Antispasmodic/ stimulates blood flow to the tissues. Repairs the	Add 10 drops of raw garlic juice to 20ml of Til oil, boil for a	Add some camphor eucalyptus oil to make it more useful.	Do not rub with too much pressure	Rasona Tail

(Contd...)

S. No.	Complaint	Green Remedies	Actions	Uses/ Dosage	Combination	Cautions	Equivalent Market Preparations
1	2	3	4	5	6	7	8
	including back strain **Specific Symptoms:** Pain due to Injury/exer –tion Swollen joints / Limbs		tissue	few minutes, filter and apply when it is luke warm. Massage gently over affected area.			
	IMPORTANT NOTICE If fracture is suspected or symptoms persist for more than a few days with-out relief – seek professional help	Arnica	Promotes healing / Antibacterial action	Soak a pad in diluted tincture and use as a compress	Take ARNIC 6X for every 2 hours	—	ARNICA Muscle oil
		Thyme	Antispas-modic, pain killer	Add 10 drops oil to 20 ml water and use as a compressor and add 5 drops of oil to a hot bath.	Add 25ml of sun flower oil for massage	—	—
		Sambhal	Analgesic / Refresher	Add 20-30 fresh leaves to a bucket of not water and use for bath.	Add eucalyptus leaves	—	Mahanarayana Tail

Head-aches

S. No.	Complaint	Green Remedies	Action	Uses and Dosage	Combination	Equivalent Market Preparations
1.	**TENSION HEAD-ACHE** May be caused by tense neck muscles due to stress. Symptoms resolve with relaxation of muscles	Ashwagandha Root	Relaxant, Tranquilizer, Analgesic	Root powder 5 gms with a cup of warm milk twice a day	Take along with Brahmi	Stresscom, (Dabur) Stressnil capsules (Baidyanath)
		Eucalyptus Oil	Relaxant / Counter irritant	Oil for application on the temples at the first hint of attack	Add drops of menthol, thymol, camphor for effective pain control.	Zandu balm, Amrutanjan, Vicks vaporub
	Specific Symptoms: Pain is usually frontal	Sunthi powdered dry rhizome Zinziber officinalis	Counter irritant	½ tsp powder well mixed in some water to make a paste, apply a thin layar on the fore head.	—	—
2.	**MIGRAINE** It is a severe form of head ache. Causes are :- food sensivity, pollution, menstrual irregularities, stress etc.	Betel Leaves leaves of Piper betel	Analgesic / Cooling	Take 2 tender leaves cut to half, fry gently in castor oil and apply on the fore head	Internally fresh tulasi juice (10ml) well-mixed in honey should be taken twice a day	Cephagran (charak) tablets 2 twice a day

S. No.	Complaint	Green Remedies	Action	Uses and Dosage	Combination	Equivalent Market Preparations
	It is associated with changes in tension within the arteries of the brain and it may last for a few minutes to several days. **Specific Symptoms:** Visual disturbances Preceding pain Pins and needles in limbs Nausea and vomiting to light sensitivity	Ajwoin Seeds Seeds of Carum roxburghianum	Analgesic	Seeds should be smoked or made in to fine powder and snuffed repeatedly to get relief.	—	1. Laghusut a sekhar pills -2 pills twice daily
		Rasna Roots Roots of Pluchex Iancelota	Anti-inflammatory analgesic	Rasna "Roots" should be made into coarse powder. This coarse powder (20 gms) should be added to 2 glasses of water. This should be kept for some time. After 30 minutes, a decoction should be prepared by keeping on the stove. ½ glass of decoction out of 2 glasses of water should be made. This ½ glass should be made into two doses, which should be taken twice a day, for 15 days	Externally If "Dasha moola coarse powder is also added, it gives faster results.	1. Maha rasnadi quatham dose 15ml + 15ml water twice a day 2. Rasnadiguggul 1 tab twice a day (Baidyanath).
3.	**NEURALGIA** Severe burning or stabbing pain	1. Eranda (castor) roots	Soothening	Pure castor oil (medicinal) 10ml,	Castor leaves.	1. Eranda tail (Dabur)

	often felt along the course of facial nerve. It may follow injury or exposure to cold.	/ oils		well mixed in a cup of warm dry ginger (sonth) decoction (one cup) should be taken twice.		
	Specific Symptoms: Severe localized pain. Related areas of skin, highly sensitive to touch.	2. Ginger (Dry – sonth) Rhizomes	Analgesic / Anti – inflammatory	—	—	2. Nagaradi Vati
		3. Vitex negundo leaves	—	For fomentation : some fresh leaves of nirgundi (Vitex Negundo) should be tied in clean cloth, this should be heated on a pan and applied on the painful parts gently for 15 minutes twice daily.	—	3. Kaisora Guggulu 2 tabs twice a day

Nervous Disorders

Ayurveda system of medicine focuses on the fitness of body, mind and spirit, often called as Holistic view. Physical manifestations of nervous disorders may include insomnia, palpitations or head aches, emotional aspects like irritability, depression, anger or guilt and lack of determination etc. reflect one's inner and spiritual vacuum.

Green herbs, plants and trees generally operate on these levels of mind-body-spirit. "Brahmi" is a good example. It is an effective blood-tonic and nerve-relaxant, taken in ghee. It is a fine brain-tonic and brings in inner calmness. Thus a single green herb works at the same time on the three vital levels—mind, body and spirit. As such most of these green remedies are wider in action comparable to modern broad-spectrum drugs.

S. No.	Problem	Green Remedies	Actions	Uses & Dosage	Combination	Equivalent Market Preparations
1.	**ANXIETY & TENSION** Stress in excess and over a long periods can lead to many complaints like anxiety and tension. The root cause being the 'cut throat' competitive environment we lieve in.	1. jatamamasi roots decoction	Mental relaxant / sedative	20ml of decoction twice a day	"Brahmi" Grutham	Serpina tabs (Himalays)
		2. Shanka Pushpi root powder	Memory booster/ mental relaxant	15ml twice a day	Sugar	Shankapushpi Syrup
	Specific Symptoms: Inability to relax, emotional instability, head aches, sleeplessness	3. Sarpa Gandha root powder.	anti-hypertension calms down/sedative	5 grams powder or tablet twice a day.	Pure ghee or water	Sarpagandha Tabs
2.	**DEPRESSION** Depression is the result of deficiency of the	1. Tulasi (Ocimum basicilcum)	Proven anti-depressant, spiritually	5ml of fresh juice of laeves twice a day.	In combinatin with honey	Tulasi tabs and syrup (Bajaj).

	nervous system	Fresh leaves	enlightens			
	Specific Symptoms: Feeling low down, misery, Lack of concentration, Lack of interest, Poor digestion, Constipation	2. Brahmi (Centala asiatica) leaves	Mental equipoiser, mild sedative, anti-depressive calms down	5ml of fresh juice extracted from tender leaves twice a day	In combination with equal quantity of pure cow ghee offers excellent results	Brahmi vati & Grutham
		3. Ashwa-Gandha (Withania somnifera roots powder	Calmposer, mental tonic, improves inner strength.	5 grams of powder twice a day	With milk or ghee	Stresscom caps (Dabur).

Blood-circulation

S. No.	Problem	Green Remedies	Actions	Uses/ Dosage	Combination	Market Preparations
1.	**POOR CIRCULATION COLD HANDS & FEET** This may be a sign of a more serious heart problem, but is often simply an inherited tendency.	Ginger Fresh juice	Circulatory stimulant, promotes warming.	5 to 10ml fresh juice thrice a day	Honey	Sunti powder 2 grams
	Specific Symptoms: Exceptionally cold hands and feet, White or 'dead' fingers (Raynaud's phenomenon)	Arjuna Bark powder of Terminalia arjuna	Strengthen circulatory system, cardio – protective.	5 grams powder well mixed in warm milk and taken twice a day	Ginger powder 2 grams	Arjun tabs (charak)
2.	**HARDENING ARTERIES** It is the outcome of the fatty deposits in blood vessels, leading to risk of strokes	1. Garlic Bulb cloves	Reduces blood cholesterol & risk of stroke	Take 1 clove twice a day	Arjun bark Powder	Garlic caps (Ranbaxy)
	Specific Symptoms: High blood pressure, blood vessel may feel hard, eye disorders. Sudden or severe pain in the legs while walking.	2. Stem of Tinospora cordifolia	-do-	5 grams powder twice a day	Garlic	Guduchi churna

Certain Common ENT Problems

S. No.	Problem	Green Remedies	Actions	Uses & Dosage	Combination	Market Drugs
1.	**EAR-ACHE** Earache is generally associated with mucous condition or infections **Specific Symptoms:** Pain, often severe, in one or both ears, Blocked sensation in the ears, Ringing sounds, Excessive waxy discharge fever, vetigo/nausea, if the inner ear is affected. **Caution:** Severe infections can lead to deafness, consult ENT surgeon.	1. Garlic : one clove of garlic should be well crushed and gently boiled in 5 tsf of gingelly oil. Filter well and instill 3 to 5 drops thrice a day, gives good results.	Analgesic/ Anti-infective Anti-bacterial/ antiseptic	3 to 5 drops thrice a day	Kanchanara guggulu or Triphala guggul 1 tab thrice a day	Rasona oil, Kshara Taila ear drops (any brand)
		2. Triphala Fine powder	Anti-inflammatory, Anti-bacterial	5 grams twice a day	With sudha guggulu 250mg twice a day.	Triphala Guggul Baidyanath, Biogest, (KAPL)
2.	**SORE THROAT** It commonly occurs due to chemical irritants inhaled or infections. It may accom	1. Turmeric + Common salt	Anti-inflammatory Anti-bacterial	As required for mouth wash, gargling	Triphalal	Turmeric pills
		2. Kanchanara	Reduces the	5 grams powder		Kanchanara

(Contd...

S. No.	Problem	Green Remedies	Actions	Uses & Dosage	Combination	Market Drugs
	pany tonsilitis, pharyngitis etc.		swelling, re moves pain	well boiled in a glass of water twice a day.		tablets
	Specific Symptoms: Pain at the back of the mouth, difficulty in swallowing, red inflamed throat, hoarseness of voice	3. Kadhira	Soothing/ Healing	Pills, chewable 3 to 4 times		Kadiradi Vati (Dabur)
		4. Triphala	Clearing/Antiseptic healthy	Powder 5 grams twice a day well mixed in hot water		Triphala Tab (Dabur)
3.	**TONSILITIS** Inflammation of the Tonsils is usually associated with infections (Bacterial/viral)	1. Kanchanara (It is the drug of choice)	Anti- inflammatory	500 mg tabs thrice a day	Hot water fomentation or gargling with salt	Kanchanara tabs (Baidyanath)
	Specific Symptoms: Severe sore throat Difficulty in swallowing Marked fever Red, enlarged tonsils, which may discharge pus. An abcess on the tonsils needs ENT consultation	2. Haridra powder	Analgesic/ Anti-bacterial	½ tsf twice a day	Tulsi decoction	Haridra Khanda (Baidynath)
		3. Tirphala+ guggulu	Heals/pain relieving	250 mg pills thrice a day	Dashamoola decoction	Septillin (Himalaya) or Biogest
4.	**MOUTH ULCERS** It is the inflammation of the mouth, resulting in redness, blisters, ulcers and submucosal	1. Triphala powder as anti-constipation	Healer/soothing	Powder 5 grams twice with hot water	Haridra 200mg tab	Triphala churna

	bleeding with pain	2. **Neem Leavs** powder	Anti-bacterial	3 grams fine powder, trice a day with water	Kadira tabs	Neem caps
	Specific Symptoms: Pain and difficulty in swallowing is the important symptom. Mild to moderate fever Foul-smell/odour from the mouth	3. **Kadira** is the choice of remedy. Take green vegetables in plenty to overcome from this	Heals the ulcers	200 mg tablets chewable 3 to 4 times a day.	Kadira oral liquid	Kadira tabs

Respiratory Complaints

S. No	Problem	Green Remedies	Actions	Uses & Dosage	Combination	Market Drugs
1.	**COUGHS** These are the most common complaints of Respiratory system. Cough is a muscle-spasm that occurs as a reaction to irritation or obstruction in the Bronchial tubes. Further, cough, often occurs in conjunction with infection like cold and flu.	1. Vasaka (Adusa) Leaves juice	Soothens/expectorant Anti-Allergic	Fresh juice or syrup preparation 10ml thrice a day	Tulasi/Pan juice	Vasaka Syrup or Oral Liq. Adusa Tabs
		2. Kantakari Powder/ Lehya	Proven-Anti-allergic, reduces esinophilic count	3 gms twice a day	Vasa	Kantakari Ghan Tabs
	Sometimes cough occurs purely due to nervous tensions	3. Banafsha Fruit/ syrup	Soothens, expectoral	syrup 10ml as required	Trijataka	Banafsha syrup
	Specific Symptoms: Wet cough may produce mucus, varying	4. Tulasi leaves juice	Anti-allergic, anti-toxin expectoral	Fresh tender leaves juice with honey as required	Pan juice/ Honey	Tulasi Cough Syrup
	from a thin, watery discharges or thick yellow or green phlegm Dry cough is an irritant in throat	5. Garlic clove	Fresh clove is anti-infectives anti-biotic.	Fresh clove a day should be taken as a preventive and 2 cloves twice a day with milk	Black pepper powder	Garlic Capsules
	Caution: In long-drawn coughs seek professional diagnosis by the experts	6. Trijataka	Proven remedy for cough.	1 to 2 tabs to be chewed as many times as required	Hot water	Trijatakadi Vati (Baidyanath)

2.	**ASTHMA** It causes repeated attacks of wheezing. These attacks produce many disabilities.	1. Vasa+ Kantakari (Lehya)	Anti-asthmatic/Anti-allergic	5gms thrice, with warm water	Pippali	Vasakantakari Avalehyam
	Specific Symptoms: Wheezing is a characteristic symptom, Cough often accompanies inability to speak, due to breathlessness, Typical difficulty in breathing out rather than breathing in.	2. Tulasi (Extract)	Expectorant Bronchodilator Antiseptic & infection	5 ml. fresh juice as required	Vasa juice offers synegistic action	Tulasi syrups, tablets
		3. Glycyrriza Glabra (yasti madhu) (root powder)	Anti inflammatory, expectorant, soothens throat	Fine powder 5 gms with warm milk thrice a day.	Vasa	Yasti pills
	Caution Severe asthma can be life-threatening and requires hospitalization.	4. Trikatu	corrects digestion, checks broncho spasm	3 gms. with warm milk	Honey	Trikatu Churna
		5. Pushkar Mool, Root powder	bronchodilator, anti-allergic, prevents hiccoughs	5 gms. powder with hot water	Honey	—

Problems of the Digestive System

S. No.	Problem	Green Remedies	Actions	Uses & Dosage	Combination	Equivalent Market Preparations
1.	**ACIDITY** It is the most prevalent health problem; if proper care is not taken, it may lead to ulcer formation in the digestive tract. Main culprit is the excessive secretion of HCl important factor of digestive juices. **Responsible Factors:** Excessive hot, spicy, fried food, cigarettes, alcohol consumption, stress-related conditions like anger, fear, worry etc. Certain drugs like pain killers, garlic hingu etc., **Key Symptoms:** Burning sensation in the chest and throat, Sour oral secretions/ belching, vomiting, headache, heaviness in the body, and lack of appetite.	1. Shatavari Root powder is the best green remedy for acidity problems	Natural Anti-acid/nutritive	3 gms. of fine powder well mixed in a cup of milk with sugar if taken twice a day works wonderfully	With milk + sugar	Swatavarex granules
		2. Amalaki Emblica officinalis) Dry fruits powder or fresh juice of fresh fruits.	Pitta Shamaka (Antiacid) Nutritive Tonic	21/2 gms. of fine powder well mixed in luke warm water, twice a day.	With sugar cane juice	Amlaki tabs (Chaitanya)
		3. Liquorice Root powder popularly known as Yasti Madhu	Soothing/ Cooling, anti-acid	2 gms. of root powder twice a day with milk.	With milk	Yasti tab (IMP COPS)

		4. Guduchi-Satva the water extract of whole plant	Anti-infective, anti-acid, immuno-modulator.	500mg of fine crystalline powder with cold water, twice a day	With cold water or honey.	Samsaman Tabs (Zandu)
		5. Ikshu Ras (Fresh-Sugar-cane juice)	Nutritive, Natural glu-cose cooling.	Fresh juice 100ml thrice a day (Note: Contraindicated in Diabetes)	Amla powder or tab	—
2.	**CONSTIPATION** Commonly it is associ-ated symptom of other diseases/problems. It is linked with poor diet/ fibreless food. Sluggish digestion or muscles tone. **Specific Symptoms:** Lack of bowel move-ments for more than 24 hours Lower abdominal dis-comfort/pain Difficulty in passing stools	(1) Triphala Fine powder	Mild laxative/ Fibrous helps in absorbing Toxins and passing out gases	5 gms. powder well dissolved in 50 ml hot water should be taken at bed time daily.	—	Triphalakada (Sandu).
		(2) Trivruth Fine Powder	Mild and safe purgation, Anti-acid Blood purifier	5 gms at bed time well dissolved in hot wate	—	Swadista Virechna churna (Zandu). Kayam Churna
		(3) Castoroil (Medici-nal)	Purgative, anti-rheumatic, Anti-inflam matory	5 to 20 ml well mixed in hot milk at bed time	—	Eranda tail (Dabur)
		(4) Isphagula seeds	Bulking Laxa-tive/Lubricates the bowel. Spe-cially useful if stools are dry in nature.	Infusion 15 ml.	—	Isphagula Churna

(Contd...

S. No.	Problem	Green Remedies	Actions	Uses & Dosage	Combination	Equivalent Market Preparations
3.	**DIARRHOEA** It is ofetn a symptom of other imbalances in the digestive system, can also be due to food poison or infections	1. Kutaja Bark powder	Good Anti-diarrhoeal/corrective	1 tab thrice a day or 3 gms powder twice a day.	Butter milk or hot water	Kutaj Tabs (Bajaj)
		2. Bilwa Fruit powder	Anti-diarrhoeal/ dysentry Anti-Amoebiasis	3 gms powder twice a day	—	Antisar Caps
	Specific Symptoms: Loose, frequent stools, Abdominal cramps or gripping pains.	3. Pudina leaves	Anti-diarrhoeal/ Anti-flatulant digestive	Fresh juice 2 tsf twice a day well mixed in honey	Honey	Pudin Hara (Dabur).
4.	**IRRITABLE BOWEL SYNDROME AND COLITIS (IBS)** It is a syndrome of multiple symptoms linked with food intolerance, anxiety or infection.	1. Kutaja bark powder	Broad-spectrum herbal Anti-infective Anti-flatulent Regulates stool formation	1 tab (250 mg) thrice a day with warm water	With Mustararista	Kutaja Tabs (DAP)
	Specific Symptoms: Bouts of diarrhoea and constipation one after the other (alternating), Bloating and gases, Mucus in stools and Dropping stools	2. Musta	Soothing/Anti-dysentric, arrest dropping of stools	Liquid 20ml thrice a day	With kutaja	Mustakarista (Baidyanath)
		3. Bilwa fruit	Strengthens digestive-organs, regulates specific in moebiasis	Halwa--5gms twice a day	Kutaja, musta	Bilwa Avalehya (Sandu)

5.	**NAUSEA & VOMITING CAUTION** Severe and prolonged vomiting requires hospitalization. It's an emergency problem.	1. Cardamom (ELA) seeds powder	Anti-nauseatic/ emetic specific for travel and morning sickness	Seeds should be chewed slowly (chewable)	—	Eladivati pills (Baidyanath)
	The common causes for nausea and vomiting are food poisoning, fevers, drugs, infections or migraine/headaches, psychological upsests.	2. Sonth (dry ginger) Rhizome powder	Specific for travel sickness, morning sickness	3 grams powder plus little sugar thrice a day	Honey	Nagara vati
		3. Tinospora (Guduchi) water extract crystals	Pacifies secretions, Anti-acid, soothens	2gms fine powder with ginger juice thrice a day	Ginger+Honey	Amritsatva
		4. Amlaki (E officials) fresh fruit juice	Anti-emetic, anti-infective, digestive appetizer	5ml fresh juice thrice a day with little honey	Honey	Vomitab syrup (charak) Madhuvari (Dabur)
6.	**LIVER PROBLEMS** In the present all round polluted background liver is the most vital organ. It's congestion is very common problem leading to may pathalogical conditions	1. Bring Raj (Ecliptalba)	Liver corrective	20ml thrice a day	Honey	Bringrajasav (Dabur)
		2. Bumyamalki small shrub with tall functions (fresh juice)	Anti-infective viral, liver protective	20ml thrice a day	Water	Nirocil tabs and syrup Nirurika caps
	Specific Symptons: Constipating tendency, bloating of abdomen, emotional liability, men-	3. Kumari	Liver--Stimulant, corrects menstrual dis-	20ml thrice a day	Warm water	Kumariasav

(Contd...

S. No.	Problem	Green Remedies	Actions	Uses & Dosage	Combination	Equivalent Market Preparations
	strual upsets, itching of palms and redness, itching eyes, poor-appetite, gradual loss of weight, Poor-sleep		orders			
		4. Triphala powder	Broad-spectrum drug to regulate the digestive apparatus.	30ml thrice a day 5gms at bed time	With warm water	Triphala Churna
		5. Haridra (Turmeric)	Liver-Protective, eliminates the toxins	5gms+Honey thrice a day	Honey	Haridra Khand (Baidyanath)
		6. Katuki powder	Liver—Corrective specific for jaundice.	2gms powder twice a day.		Jaundex. Syrup (Sandu)

Urinary Problems

Introduction

The kidneys and urinary system often measure one's health status, since it is the excretory channel engaged in removing the toxins from the system.

Herbal/green remedies usually include some urinary antiseptic. Soothing and tender herbs are included in the drugs to reduce inflammation and repair damage to the mucous membranes and diuretics to increase the flow of urine to flush out toxins and other unwanted materials like dead bacteria etc.

These green remedies always take care of the living system by taking away the toxins from the body and giving in the vital factors required for the human system's porper functioning.

Urinary Problems

S. No.	Problem	Green Remedies	Action	Uses & Dosage	Combination	Market Drugs
1.	**UTI & CYSTITIS** Infections of the urinary tract generally lead to cystitis in women and 'urethritis' in men. In some instances, the kidneys are also affected. **Specific Symptoms:** Frequent, painful urination, Blood, mucus or pus in urine, fever, pain anywhere from the groin to the mid-back. **Caution:** consult an urologist, if symptoms are severe and persistant.	1. Gokshura (Whole plant extract)	Anti-infective, Diuretic, strengthens Urinary system	Whole plant ex tract 20ml twice a day	Triphala guggulu 250mg	Gokshura guggulu (sandu)
		2. Chandana sandal wood Heart wood	Cooling/ sedative promotes urination anti-bacterial	Wood pills 200 mg	Gokshura	Chandanadi vati
		3. Usheera Roots decoction	Cooling/ stimulates urine	20ml twice	Guduchi	Usheerasav
		4. Guduchi (Whole plant powder)	Balances all the doshas specific urinary anti septic	5gms powder with milk twice a day	Gokshura guggulu	Amrita satva

(Contd...

S. No.	Problem	Green Remedies	Actions	Uses & Dosage	Combination	Market Drugs
2.	**URINARY STONES** Deposits of insoluble material—usually calcium salts—which can be associated with changes in the acidity or alkalinity of the urine	1. Pashanabhedi—Specific for stones (whole plant extract)	Specific for urinary stones, it breaks and dissolves the stones	Decoction 20ml thrice a day.	Chandraprabha	Cystone Tabs
	Specific Symptoms: Sensation of burning while urinating blood in the urine Severe pain between loin and groin	2. Gokshura	-do-	-do-	-do-	Gokshura guggulu Tab
		3. Shilajit	-do-	Powder, caps 250mg	Gokshur	Shilajit Caps
3.	**PROSTATE PROBLEMS** It may be due to aging or infection of the prostate gland	1. Chandana Heart wood powder	Diuretic/Anti infective strengthens urinary system	5gms twice a day		Chandraprabhavati
	Specific Symptoms: Difficulty in urinating, dribbling Urine retention in severe cases	2. Gokshura Whole plant	Diuretic/Anti inflammatory	20ml decoction twice daily	Chandana	Gokshura Kada
		3. Shilajit powder	Specific reduces prostate elargement	caps 250 mg twice a day	Chandana	Shilajit Caps
		4.Kanchanara	Anti-inflammatory	tabs-250 mg twice a day		Kanchanara Tabs

Female Complaints

S. No.	Problem	Green Remedies	Actions	Uses & Dosage	Combination	Equivalent Market Preparations
1.	**PAINFUL MENSTRUATION** Moderate to severe pain during the menstruation	Kumari [Aloe] Leaf pulp juice	Uterine Sedative	In painful menstruation 4 to 6 tea spoon full of fresh leaf pulp juice thrice a day offers prompt relief	Saracá indica bark-decoction 20ml	Kumaryasav Oral liquid
2.	**IRREGULAR PERIODS**	1. Kumar (Aloe barbadensis) **Preparation** Remove skin of 3 leaves, collect the pulp and put pulp into a brass vessel and boil till it becomes thick and brownish colour.	Uterine/Tonic regulator	Rub the prepared brown paste on a clean stone. Tea spoon full of tulsi paste should be taken twice a day for 7 days before the menstruation	Ashoka, nimba	Kumaryasav Oral liquid
		2. Neem (Nimba)- Azadirachta Indica Bark-Hot infusion	—	30ml. decoction thrice a day for 7 days.	Ashoka, Kumari	—

(Contd...

S. No.	Problem	Green Remedies	Actions	Uses & Dosage	Combination	Equivalent Market Preparations
3.	**EXCESSIVE PERIODS**	1. Vasa/ Adoosa Leaves juice	Stops bleeding	Fresh juice derived from 5 to 10 leaves twice a day with honey	Amla powder	Vasa Tabs
		2. Shatavari Tubers juice	Uterine sedative	4 tea spoon full of juice or 5 gms of powder thrice a day with salt.	Vasa	Shatavari Churna
		3. Nagakesara Flowers powder	Uterine sedative	—	—	Nagakesara Churna
4.	**WHITE DISCHARGE (Leucorrhoea)**	1. Kumari (Aloe) Pulp juice	Uterine Cleanser	30ml thrice a day	Ashoka	Kumari Asav
		2. Shatavari Turbers Powder	—	5 grams twice with milk. 10ml with honey, rice wash	Dashamoola	Shatavari Churna
		3. Guduchi Leaves juice	—			Guduchi Satva
5.	**MENOPAUSAL SYNDROME** In most women, the menopausal change occurs without any unpleasant symptoms, the only change being the	1. Milk is a rich source of calcium and vit-D. since these get de-	—	—	—	—

	stoppage of menstrual flow. However in some others, many disturbing changes take place like:- Hot flushes and night sweats, Vaginal dryness, Increased facial hair dryness of the skin of the body.	pleted around menopause, a good quantity of milk should be given				
		2. Liquorice popularly known as Yastimadhu or meeta lakdi is a natural source of female hormone-oestrogen-this can be used with milk.	Natural female hormone supplement	1 tsf twice a day with 1 glass of milk	Ashwagandha or Brahmi	Yasti Tabs
	Special Note : Women should not worry too much about becoming old or loosing beauty as these are natural changes.	Ashwagandha is also useful to reduce irritation and strain	Calms down the emotional problems associated with menopause.	5gms twice a day with mik	Brahmi	Stress win Caps (Baidyanath)
6.	**INFERTILITY (Female)** If a woman has not con-	Bark of Banyan tree	—	10 grams of powder should be taken early morn-	Dashamoola quatham should be used	Panchavalkala Churna

(Contd...

S. No.	Problem	Green Remedies	Actions	Uses & Dosage	Combination	Equivalent Market Preparations
	ceived even after one to two years after natural intercourse with her husband, then there are chances of `Fertility' problems, she may not be producing eggs, or her fallopian tubes may be blocked etc.	The fresh bark of Banyan tree dried enough to make powder should be taken.		ing for 60 days	alongwith these medicines	
7.	**FATIGUE** Because of heavy work for prolonged time, or excessive mental activity, one experiences fatigue, tiredness, slight giddines, body pains and other vague symptoms	1. Any fresh fruit juice helps a lot in such conditions	1 glass	—	—	—
		2. Fresh Grape juice is extremely useful	1 glass	—	—	—
		3. Dates or (Kharjura) are great source of instant energy.	4 to 5	With milk	—	—
		4. Ashwagandha roots powder can be taken regularly.	5 gms daily at bed time	With milk	—	Stressnil

Foot-problems

Even though we use our feet and legs for every kind of movement of life, unfortunately these are mostly neglected organs of our body. We notice them only when there is a serious problem affecting our every day movement. All such important problems and their remarks are enumerated below.

General Care:

1. Keep the leg and foot always clean. Even when there is a minor cut or boil take proper care.
2. Always apply pure coconut oil over the soles of the feet and on legs, preferably before going to bed. Coconut oil is a good nutritive, as well as lubricating agent. It nourishes and keeps skin intact. Even though this daily oil massage appears to be a very simple one, in the long run this practice offers excellent results by preventing varicose veins, cramps, cuts, corns etc.
3. Avoid very tight shoes and other foot wear. Soften new pairs of chappals with some lubricants so that there is no friction or pressure on your feet.
4. Legs and feet bear our weight constantly as we are always on them; try to provide them the much needed rest in between working hours.

S. No.	Problem	Green Remedies	Action	Use & Doses	Combinations	Equivalent Market Preparations
1.	**VARICOSE VEINS** Swollen or stretched veins in the legs, associated with poor venous return or raised abdominal pressure as in obesity, pregnancy or chronic constipation. **Specific Symptoms:** Visible, enlarged and stretched veins – "Blue – veins", Pain in the legs	Castor Oil (luke warm)	Mild analgesic / Anti-inflammatory / lubricant	Lukewarm – castor oil should be applied over the varicose veins daily for 40 days, then repeat on alternate days.	Triphala guggulu pills, 2 pills twice a day with warm water	1.Eranda taila (Dabur) 2. Triphala guggulu

(Contd...

S. No.	Problem	Green Remedies	Action	Use & Doses	Combinations	Equivalent Market Preparations
2.	**WARTS** Small, hard growth in the outer layer of the skin, due to a virus generally found on the palms and soles	1. Garlic (bulb) crushed, for external application	Analgesic/ Anti-inflammatory Anti-Viral	Cruch 2 to 3 cloves or more according to the size and apply twice a day preferably at bed time.	Spread a thin bandage over the corn and apply moderate heat after application of medicines	1. Garlic Pearls (Internal) 2. Corn Cap dressing.
	Specific Symptoms: hard growth with pain	Castor Oil	Lubricant	Daily application softens the corn	—	—
		Garlic Oil/ Lemon Oil	Analgesic & Lubricant	—	—	—
3.	**CRACKED SKIN OF PALM & SOLE** It is a very common problem of the people exposed to detergents, agricultural operations, unclean and soap water	Utmost cleanliness of the plan and soles should be maintained		—	—	—
	Specific Symptoms: Visible skin crackes over the plams of hands and soles of the feet, with swelling and pain, some times even pus is formed due to infections	1. Manjista Powder (Rubia Cordifolia)	Healing Antiseptic	5. grams of powder twice a day.	Castor Oil	Pinda Tailam Oil for application is a good remedy
		2. Triphala Powder	Healing /cleaning/ Analgesic	20 gms powder boiled in 1 liter of water, should be poured into a clean vessel, hands and feet should be well immersed for 30 minutes before going to bed. Then external oils/ointments as indicated should be applied over the affected parts.	Manjista Powder	—

Skin — Herbal Approach

Green remedies recommended for skin problems / care are meant for restoring internal balance using cooling / cleansing herbs are better than creams that may alleviate symptoms but do nothing in the healing.

Excessive pitta dosha causes blood vitiation, thereby causes skin problems. Similarly too much vata results in dry, rough skin, while excess kapha dosha leads to weeping or oozing skin conditions.

Skin

S. No.	Problem	Green Remedies	Actions	Uses/ Dosage	Combination	Market Preparations
1.	**ECZEMA** It is an inflammatory condition of skin, some times localized, appearing like 'bark of the tree'.	1. Neem Leaves decoction leaves of Azadirachta indica	For clearing the patches	Anti-bactierial Anti-septic	As required should be poured over the patches	Nimbadi Churna
		2. Kutaja Bark powder of Holarrhena antidysen-terica	Anti Itching / soothing / healing	250mg tablets made from pure bark powder thrice a day	Manjista / Amlaki Kutaja tabs	Kutaja Ghana Vati
	Specific Symptoms: Red, inflamed patches Itching Certain types are oozing, forming crusts of serum Lesions may bleed in acute conditions	3. Yastimadhu Root powder of Glycyrr-hiza glasra	Anti-inflammatory	3 grams powder twice a day.		Yasti Powder
		4. Brahmi Powder Leaves of Bacopa Monnieri	Anti bacterial/ Anti septic			Brahmivati, Bivita Tab (DAP)

(Contd...

S. No.	Problem	Green Remedies	Actions	Uses/ Dosage	Combination	Market Preparations
2.	**ACNE** Inflammation of the sebaceous glands in the skin, which may start with blackheads. It is usually common in the teenage population. **Specific Symptoms:** Inflamed pustules Excess oily facial skin Infected cysts and scarring in severe cases	1. Garlic Bulb	Antibacterial anti fungal, good antiseptic indicated in infected skin	Rub, the affected area with a cut clove of garlic daily twice.	Turmeric	Garlic capsules (Ranbaxy)
		2. Cabbage	Anti-bacterial / Nutritive / Healing	Extract fresh juice and apply over the affected area		
		3. Turmeric Paste of Curcuma longa	Anti-bacterial / improves complexion	Apply the paste	Sandal wood	Vicco Turmeric Cream
		4. Sandal Wood Paste of Santalum album	Cooling / promotes healing / complexion	Apply the paste	Turmeric	
3.	**PSORIASIS** A disturbed skin condition resulting from the over production of skin-keratinocytes, which fail to mature into normal keratine. It may be due to immune dysfunction or infection /allergies/ over	1. Kutaja Bark powder	Specific for psoriasis anti-itching	Bark powder tablets. 200 mg thrice a day	Neem caps with ghee mixed milk	Kutaj Tabs (DAP)
		2. Neem Oil	Anti bacterial/ Itching	5ml oil well mixed in a glass of milk twice a day	Brahmi Tab	Neem Caps (Phytopharma)

	stress worry. A tendency of psoriasis often runs in families.	3. Manjista Bark powder of Rubia cordifolia	Blood purifier	15ml decoction twice a day	Gooseberry powder	Manjistarista
	Specific Symptoms & Signs: Patches of red skin, often with silver – coloured scales Cycle of remission and recurrence	4. Khadira heart wood of Acacia catechu	Specific drug for Psoriasis	Khadira powder decoction 15ml twice a day	Gooseberry Powder	Khadira liquid
4.	**FUNGAL INFECTIONS** Ring worm infections are caused by fungi. The toes and the scalp are the most commonly affected areas	1. Aloe pulp of Aloevera	Cooling / demulcent Anti parasitic, useful in scabies	Apply gel from fresh leaf		Kumari Asav
	Specific Symptoms: Red, irritated patches Peeling or scaly skin Itching	2. Sariba bark of Desmodium gangeticum	-do-	Fresh decoction of sariba bark 20 ml thrice a day		Sariba Tabs (Baidyanath)
		3. Neem Leaves paste	Anti parasatic fungal	Fresh paste to apply	Turmeric powder	Neem Based oil

Hair

S. No.	Problem	Green Remedies	Action	Uses/ Doseage	Combination	Market Preparations
1.	**ALOPECIA HAIR LOSS** In this, hair loss may be total or patchy, mild loss can be due to vitamin deficiency	1. (Bringaraj) Eclipta Alba hair oil of leaves	Improves hair growth, strengthens the hair	Apply on head & massage over the patches twice a day	Gooseberry	Bhringraj hair oil
	Specific Symptoms: Bald patches or loose hair	2. Arnica flowers	Stimulates blood circulation	Apply as cream or ointment	Vitamin supplements	Arinica oil
		3. Gooseberry Fruit pulp powder	Nutritive, natural vitamin 'C'	Externally apply as oil Internally as powder 5 gms twice a day	Bhringraj	Hair Rich Oil (Capro)
2.	**PREMATURE GREYING**	Same remedies are recommended				
3.	**DANDRUFF** Small flakes of dead skin on the scalp. It may be accompanied by seborrhoeic dermatitis. Obvious deposit on collars Hair dry and brittle, or greasy with yellow flakes.	1. Ritha nuts 2. Sikkakai 3. Amla ki fruit pulp 4. Neem leaves 5. Henna leaves	Cleansing and anti-inflammatory, rich in saponins	Soak in water and apply Readymade preparations	Gooseberry	Ritha Powder Kunthala Herbal shampoo (Green Valley)

The Green Remedies and Their Medicinal Applications

Green Herbs	Useful in Diseases	Important Medicinal Applications
1. **Ajamoda**	(a) Hiccough (b) Colic (c) Abdominal distension (d) Aruchi (e) Worm infestation (f) Appetizer (g) Bronchitis (h) Asthma (i) Intestinal disorders	**Gastric discomfort** Take 1 tsp fine powder of ajamoda with luke warm water, this relieves from gastric discomfort within minutes.
2. **Akarakarabha**	(a) Swelling (b) Sore throat (c) Fevers (d) Increases male erections	**Sore throat** In sore throat little bit of akarakarabha fine powder well mixed in honey, if applied as throat paint inside the oral cavity gives prompt relief.
3. Amalaki-Cooling	(a) Fever (b) Diabetes (c) Jaundice (d) Daha burning sensation/ acidity (e) Skin problems (f) Rejuvenator/tonic (g) Vertigo	Eat fresh amalaki a day for 40 days during Dec-Jan of every year, be disease free for a year.
4. **Arjuna Twak**	(a) Bleeding (b) Diabetic wounds (c) Obesity (d) Cardio-protective (e) Heart protective (f) Controls mild B.P.	**Weight control** Obese people should take 5 grams i.e., 1 tsp powder of Arjuna, well mixed in luke warm water daily, once for 40 days. It reduces the fat and weight. Further, it safeguards the heart, kidney. This cycle should be repeated as required.

5. **Ashoka (Saraca Indica)**	(a) Dysmenorrhoea (b) Worms (c) Visha (d) Blood Disorders	**A boon to the ladies** Ashoka bark powder 15 grams added to 200ml water, should be boiled till it reduces to 50 ml. This should be filtered & used twice a day in 2 divided doses (each dose 25ml). It regulates the menstrual cycle disturbances, dysmenorrhoea
6. **Ashwagandha (Withania Somnifer)**	(a) Consumption/General debility (b) Vitiligo (c) Oligospermia (d) Infertility (e) Aphrodasiac	**Most useful application-white patches** 1. In Vitiligo (Leucoderma) popularly identified as white patches 5 grams of powder of Ashwagandha. Twice a day for 3 months gives good results. 2. In run-down conditions 5 grams of powder well boiled in 200ml of milk should be taken at night. It rebuilds the system.
7. **Ashwatha**	(a) Fractures (b) Vomiting (c) Burns (d) Inflammation of mouth (mukhapaka) (e) Ear diseases (f) A female infertility	**Oral-wash** Ashwatha bark decoction is a wonderful mouth wash, it removes bad smell from the mouth and pacifies even acute stomatitis, non responsive to **conventional therapy**-Prepare decoction of 15 gms bark coarse powder mixed to 200ml of water, reduce it to 50ml. Use it in gargle twice a day.
8. **Bala**	(a) Rheumatism (b) Fevers	—

	(c) Consumption (d) Painful conditions	
9. **Bhallataka**	(a) Piles (b) Dysentery (c) Worms (d) Asthma (e) Vitiligo	**Caution** Poisonous—drug to be used under medical supervision after proper purification only.
10. **Brahmi (Centella Asiatica)**	(a) Skin Diseases (b) Anaemia (c) Bleeding (d) Metabolic disorders (e) Memory booster	For **Good memory**—Two fresh leaves after cleaning under running water should be crushed with little bit of sugar and chewed by the school going children in early morning. It is a natural memory booster
11. **Bhringaraja (Eclipta Alba)**	(a) Swelling (b) Anaemia (c) Skin disorders (d) Heart diseases (e) Jaundice	**For black & lustrous hair** It is a reputed hair tonic, arrests the grey hair and promotes the hair growth. It can be used as a regular hair oil instead of coconut oil. Regular application brings in many benefits.
12. **Chandana (Sandal Wood)**	(a) Fatigue (b) Consumption/general debility (c) Leucorrhoea (d) Burning sensation (e) Urinary disorders (f) Prickly heat	Make 1 tsf sandal wood paste on a stone by adding a little bit of water and 1/2 tsf of sugar and stir well. This should be consumed daily in the afternoon to solve the burning urination and burning sensation of the body especially during summer. It is a wonderful home remedy
13. **Chitrakmool**	(a) Swelling (b) Piles	**Caution** Roots of chitrakmool are

	(c) Consumption/general debility (d) Anaemia	highly potent, they can cause abortion when taken in high doses.
14. Dadima (Punica Granatum)	(a) Fever (b) Amavata/Arthritis (c) Vomiting sensation (d) Vertigo (e) Dysentery (f) It can also be used as antidote for "Bhang" intoxication	In **morning sickness** of the pregnant women crush, fruit pulp of dadima and extract fresh juice by pressing over a filter cloth. Take 1 cup of the juce every morning on empty stomach. This resolves morning sickness.
15. Daruharidra	(a) Fevers (b) Erysipelis (c) skin Allergy (d) Urinary problem	—
16. Devadaru	(a) Swelling (b) Hiccough (c) Diabetes (d) Fever (e) Bleeding (f) Cold (g) Cough	—
17. Dhanyaka	(a) Fever (b) Burning sensation (c) Vomiting (d) Cough (e) Piles (f) Worms	**In burning urination** Dhanyaka (Coriandrum sativum); whole plant is useful in burning urine problems. Crush fresh plant and obtain juice. This should be taken orally in the dose of 3 teaspoonfull with some honey thrice a day. It is a pleasant way of resolving burning urination.
18. Draksha (Dry)	(a) Sore throat (b) Jaundice (c) Consumption	One of the most useful application is in constipation, 2 to 3 dried grapes

	(d) Bleeding (e) Burning sensation (f) Sleeplessness (g) Urinary problems (h) Diabetes (i) Anaemia	(munakka) should be soaked in a glass of water over night. One should consume these swollen dried fruits on empty stomach daily. This will resolve the constipating tendency in a sweeter way.
19. Ela	(a) Urinary disorders (b) Pain (c) Itching (d) Thirst (e) Bad odour in mouth, dry cough (f) Vomiting sensation	**Travel sickness** Ela 2 fruits should be crushed duly removing outer layer and well mixed in honey. 1 tsf should be taken orally before one hour of the travel in bus/train/flight. This effectively arrests travel sickness problem.
20. Eranda Tailam	(a) Swelling (b) Fevers (c) Amavata/Arthritis (Rheumatoid) (d) Constipation	**Corn** Regular application of castor oil over the corns makes them soft and painless over a longer time, this solves the corn problems.
21. Gokshuru	(a) Rheumatism (b) Urinary disorders (c) Urinary Stones (d) Swelling (e) Impotence	Gokshura is a natural drug for male erection problems especially resulting after excessive use of modern drugs. Fine powder of whole plant (dried) in the dose of 5 gms twice a day with a cup of warm milk helps a lot.
22. Guggulu	(a) Tumours (b) Glands (c) Swellings (d) Piles (e) Worms (f) Arthritis (g) Obesity	Punched guggulu with triphala is an effective way of combating the elevated cholesterol level without any side effect but with benefits like weight control etc.

	(h) Anti-cholesterol (i) Painful condition	
23. Guduchi	(a) Burning sensation (b) Anaemia (c) Jaundice (d) Skin Disease (e) Gout (f) Fevers (g) Worms (h) Syphilis (i) Rheumatism (j) Rejuvenative/tonic	**Chronic & unknown fevers** Tinospora cordifolia (Guduchi) is a green creeper of choice in chronic fevers, creeper of unknown origin. Fresh juice of 5 leaves plus 1 tsf of pure honey thrice a day for 40 days should be given before 1 hour of meals time. Drastically cures all fevers.
24. Hareetaki (Harda)	(a) Swelling (b) Fever (c) Constipation (d) Indigestion (e) Diabetes (f) Eye diseases (g) Diarrhoea (h) Dysentery	**Indigestion** Remove seed and crush the fruit bark of harda (Terminalia chebula). One should chew little bit of this fruit bark with some jaggery 15 minutes before food. It resolves indigestion problem.
25. Haridra	(a) Skin Disease (b) Itching (c) Diabetic wounds (d) Worms (e) Cold (f) Sore throat (g) Swelling (h) Complexion-promoter (i) Respiratory allergy (j) Skin Allergy	In severe cold and respiratory allergy-one should regularly inhale haldi duly kept on slow fire for 5 minutes twice a day. It gives relief.
26. Hingu	(a) Abdominal discomfort (b) Gulma (c) Worms (d) Cough (e) Catarch (cold) (f) Bronchitis	**Colic pain** Hingu should be fried in ghee and made into powder. 1/2 to 1 tsf of this should be taken with first bolous of food, well mixed with cow's

	(g) Dysmenorrhoea (h) Asthma (i) Indigestion (j) Colic (k) Hysteria (l) Ear diseases	ghee.
27. Ikshuraka	(a) Male sterility/ impotence (b) Swelling (c) Kidney stones/urinary diseases (d) Thirst (e) Eye disorders (f) Gout (g) Gonorrhoea (h) Ascities (i) Liver diseases	**In Jaundice** Plenty of sugarcane juice with some lemon juice should be taken. It cleans the system by promoting urination and relieves thirst. It is also good nutritive.
28. Jatiphala	(a) Throat diseases (b) Diarrhoea & Dysentery (c) Prameha/excessive urination (d) Male sterility/impotence (e) Abdominal distension (f) Indigestion (g) Colic (h) Vomiting/nausea (i) Headache (j) Rheumatism (k) Discolouration of face/ leprotic ulcers.	**Hyper pigmented patches/ discolouration** : Rub the jatiphala fruit with water and apply on the dicoloured patches, keep till it dries and then wash off. Apply continuously for 1 week to 10 days to get good results.
29. Jatipatri	(a) Cosmetic/to promote facial complexion. (b) Vomiting (c) Asthma (d) Thirst (e) Worm infestation	—

30. Jatamansi	(a) Visarpa (b) As a cosmetic/white hair/grey hair (c) Brain tonic (d) Hysteria (e) Epilepsy (f) Skin disorders (g) Kushta (h) Promotes sleep	**Safe sedative** Jatamansi decoction is a good herbal sedative in disturbed sleep conditions due to stress and strain of every day problems.
31. Jeeraka—Cumin Cyminum	(a) Nervine (b) Uterine disorders (c) Fever (d) Male imp/sterility (e) Fatigue (f) Eye disorders (g) Abdominal distention (h) Vomiting (i) Diarrhoea/dysentery (j) Paralysis (k) Hiccough (with honey/ jaggery)	**Good digestive** 5 gms cleaned jeera, added to 100ml of pure water and boiled till it is reduced to 25ml. Filter and use as a single dose. Little sugar can be added if desired. It is digestive, expels gas, promotes appetite and well being by removing ill-feelings of abdominal discomfort.
32. Kachoram	(a) Cough (b) Fevers (c) Aromatic (can be added to bath water)	**Aromatic bath** Add 5 grams of powder to a bucket full of hot water and keep for a while then have a bath. It offers pleasant sensation because it has rich aroma which removes bad body order.
33. Kantakari	(a) Asthma/bronchial diseases (b) Cough (c) Fever (d) Heart diseases (e) Esnophilia (f) Bronchitis (g) Sleeplessness (h) Fevers	**Karpoora taila (oil)** Pain oil. A good pain oil can be prepared by adding 10gms of pure karpoor crystals to 100ml of til oil, heat gently for 10 minutes. When it is lukewarm apply and massage on the painful joints, parts, head etc. It is

	(i) Prickly heat (j) Itch (k) Leucorrhoea (l) Gonorrhoea (m) Toothache (n) Headache	an effective home remedy.
34. Katukarohini	(a) Bleeding (b) Burning sensation. (c) Fevers (d) Worms (e) Liver diseases / jaundice	**In Jaundice** Katuki is a well proven liver corrective. 1 gram of this powder well mixed in 5 gms of Amla churna, can be taken twice a day in jaundice for 7 days. It offers excellent results.
35. Khadira	(a) Itching (b) Cough (c) Toothache (d) Obesity (e) Worms (f) Diabetes (g) Fevers (h) Vitiligo (i) Anaemia (j) Skin disorders (k) Syphilis (l) Diarrhoea (b) Dysentery (c) Bleeding disorders (d) Throat ulcers	**In mouth & throat ulcers** Khadiradi vati pills—available in the Ayurvedic shops, prepared from Khadira, if chewed 3 to 4 times a day clears the ulcers of mouth, throat. This should be continued for 15 days in chronic conditions.
36. Kiratatikta	(a) Fevers (b) Asthma / Bronchial disorders (c) Bleeding disorders (d) Burning sensation (e) Cough (f) Swelling (g) Thirst (h) Skin diseases (i) Worms	**Anti-malarial** Decoction made from kirata tikta is a good remedy for malaria and other chronic fevers. It is very bitter in taste, sometimes may cause vomiting.

37. Krishna Jeeraka	(a) Jwara (b) Cold catarrh (c) Worms (d) Diarrhoea (e) Dymenerrhoea	—
38. Kumari	(a) Fatigue worms (b) Male impotency (c) Liver diseases (d) Eye diseases (e) Constipation (f) Fevers (g) Burns (h) Prickly heat (i) Skin diseases	**In liver disorders** Crush a fresh leaf pulp of aloe barbadensis, take 2 tsf juice well mixed with pure honey twice a day before meals. It takes care of your liver.
39. Kushta	(a) Male infertility / impotence (b) Gout (c) Visarpa (d) Cough (e) Skin diseases (f) Rheumatism (g) Swelling (h) Obesity (i) Headache (j) Eczema (k) Asthma (l) Hysteria (j) Epilepsy	—
40. Kutaja Twak (Bark)	(a) Piles (b) Bleeding disorders (c) Thirst (d) Kustha /Skin diseases (e) Diarrhoea / Dysentery	**Kutaja for old & fevers** Roast seeds of kutaja and grind to fine powder. Add ½ tsf of powder into 1 cup of tea and cunsume twice daily for 7 days. This cures cold and fevers.
41. Laksha	(a) Cosmetic (b) Hiccough	Powder of laksha is useful in bleeding conditions, 2

	(c) Cough (d) Fevers (e) Visarpa (f) Worms (g) Skin diseases (h) Blood diseases (i) Uterine diseases (j) Anaemia	grams of the powder well mixed in butter taken twice a day stops bleeding from the gums and piles.
42. Piper Cubeba	(a) Sore throat (b) Indigestion (c) Gonorrhoea (d) Bronchitis	—
43. Lavanga	(a) Eye Diseases (b) Male impotence (c) Colic pains (d) Headache (e) Toothache (f) Cold (g) Throat diseases (h) Liver diseases (i) Bronchitis	**Head-ache** Take one or two cloves and rub on the stone by adding few drops of water to make a fine paste. This paste can be applied on the forehead for prompt relief of head-ache. The same paste can be used as regular application over the painful teeth for pain management.
44. Lodhra	(a) Eye disease (b) Diarrhoea / dysentery (c) Leucorrhoea (d) Bleeding disorders (e) Skin diseases	**A good female tonic** 'Lodhrasava' an oral liquid medicine chiefly derived from bark of lodhra tree is a proven female tonic especially useful in white discharge, menstrual pain etc.
45. Madhusnuhi	(a) Constipation (b) Abdominal discomfort (c) Colic (d) Epilepsy (e) Pain (f) Syphilis (g) Chronic Rheumatism	—

46. Manjistha	(a) Cosmetic uses (b) Throat diseases (c) Swelling (d) Eye diseases (e) Ear diseases (f) Dysentery (g) Skin diseases (h) Visarpa (i) Diabetes	A proven blood purifier—Manjista is a well proven drug for all skin problems like eczema, blood disorders, itching etc. It purifies the blood and boosts up the facial complexion. A good beauty aid. It is available at the Ayurvedic stores as Maha manjistarist, 15ml of this Liquid with equal quantity of water should be taken twice a day.
47. Maricha	(a) Asthma /Bronchial diseases (b) Colic (c) Worms (d) Syphilis (e) Fevers (f) Diarrhoea (g) Indigestion (h) Abdominal discomfort (i) Cough (j) Cold (k) Heart diseases (l) Headache (m) Skin diseases	**Cold-prone people** 'Maricha'–the black pepper powder indicated in cold-prone people. They should use fine powder well mixed with warm rice and ghee regularly during meals. In Sinusitis, black pepper fine powder well mixed in some jaggery and sweet curd should be taken for relief.
48. Musta (Cyperus Rotundus)	(a) Thirst (b) Fevers (c) Worms (d) Burning sensation (e) Jaundice (f) Diarrhoea	**A good pediatric anti-diarroheal** Prepare the decoction of coarse powder of tubers of musta, to 10 ml of this liquid well mixed with honey can be given to children to stop the watery and loose motions effectively.
49. Nagakesara	(a) Itching (b) Swelling	**Bleeding piles** In summer when bleeding

	(c) Veneral diseases (d) Bleeding piles (e) Dysentry (f) Leucorrhoea (g) Indigestion	takes place form the piles, 3gms of fine powder of Nagakesara should be well mixed in 5 grams of fresh butter and cunsumed twice a day. It promptly checks the bleeding tendency.
50. Nimba	(a) Vomiting (b) Skin diseases (c) Diabetes (d) Gout (e) Warts (f) Gonorrhoea (g) Fevers	**In burning stomach** Crush the neem bark into about 4″ × 4″ piece and keep it in a cup of hot water for 20 minutes then strain. One should take this one cup hot infusion twice a day for 7 days. Burning is resolved naturally.
51. Nirgundi	(a) Colic (b) Indigestion (c) Fevers (d) Worms (e) Rheumatism (f) Painful joints (g) Pain (h) Spleen disease (i) Sleeping disorders	One can use the fresh leaves of nirgundi for fomentation as well as hot water bath to ward off painful conditions of joints and body.
52. Parpateka	(a) Blood diseases (b) Fevers (c) Thirst (d) Burning sensation (e) Gonorrhoea (f) Vomiting	—
53. Patola	(a) Itching (b) Skin diseases (c) Fever (d) Burning sensation	—

54. Pippali	(a) Thirst (b) Fever (c) Intestinal diseases (d) Consumption (e) Ascites (f) Piles (g) Abdominal diseases	**A good vehicle for drug** Ayurveda recommends pippali churna as an effective vehicle for drug delivery. Generally it is used in powder form well mixed in honey. 2 grams is the usual dose.
55. Punarnava: (Salt Free Diet)	(a) Swelling (b) Anaemia (c) Heart diseases (d) Cough (e) Blood disorders (f) Colic (g) Urinary diseases (h) Eye diseases (i) Rheumatism (j) Fevers	**A good leafy curry** Fresh leaves curry is generally recommended in the swelling of feet, face etc. It improves the kidney function to flush-out the accumulated toxins through urine.
56. Rakta Chandana	(a) Vomiting (b) Thirst/Burning sensation (c) Bleeding disorders (d) Eye diseases (e) Male impotency/ sterility (f) Fevers (g) Toxic conditions (h) Skin diseases	**Face pack** Red sandal wood is almost included in every herbal face packs in combination with other herbs. Even it can be singularly used as face pack to prevent summer effects mixed in cold milk.
57. Rasna	(a) Gout (b) Cough (c) Swellings (d) Abdominal distention (e) Sore throat (f) Sciatica (g) Hydrocele (h) Hernia (i) Rheumatism	**Caution** Rasna is a proven drug for arthritis, however it should not be taken by the people prone to piles, acidity and bleeding as it may aggravate.

58. Rasona	(a) Male sterility/ impotency (b) Cosmetic (c) Nervine (d) Eye diseases (e) Heart diseases (f) Fevers (g) Cough (h) Colic (i) Constipation (j) Swelling (k) Piles (l) Skin diseases (m) Worms (n) Asthma/Bronchial diseases (o) Dysmenorrhoea (p) Ear diseases (q) Hysteria	**Blood pressure regulator** Remove the outer cover of one garlic clove, crush and soak in butter milk for one hour and take this paste once in a day. It regulates the blood pressure. People with 'Hot' temperament should not take this as it is hot in nature.
59. Shalamali	(a) Impotency (b) Spermatorrhoea (c) Diarrhoea (d) Bleeding disorders (e) Burning Sensation (f) Spleenic diseases	**Bleeding disorders** The resin obtained from the shalmali tree is used in the dose of 1 1/2-2 gms with honey to arrest any type of bleeding.
60. Shariba	(a) Male disorders/ Impotecy (b) Indigestion (c) Asthma/Breathing disorders (d) Cough (e) Bleeding diseases (f) Fevers (g) Diarrhoea (h) Syphilis/Gonorrhoea (i) Burning sensation (j) Epilepsy (k) Skin diseases/Leprosy (l) Itching	**A sweety summer drink** 'Sariba panam' a syrup based preparation of sariba should be taken as summer drink to get relief from thirst, burning sensation etc. It is a proven blood purifier. Dose: 30ml well mixed in 100ml of cold water once or twice a day.

61. **Sharkara (Sugar)**	(a) Vomiting (b) Fainting (c) Thirst (d) Burning sensation (e) Bleeding disorders (f) Male diseases/ Impotency	Usually used as a vehicle for the medicines.
62. **Shatavari**	(a) Nervine (b) Eye diseases (c) Diarrhoea (d) Male impotency/ sterility (e) Bleeding disorders (f) Swelling (g) Epilepsy (h) Consumption	**White discharge (leucorrhoea)** Crush tubers of asparagus racemosus i.e. shatavari to obtain fresh juice. Consume 5 tsf fresh juice on empty stomach in the early morning and evening for 15 days. It arrests the discharge and bad odour.
63. **Shunthi**	(a) Male impotency (b) Swelling (c) Asthma/breathing diseases (d) Anaemia (e) Filariasis (f) Intestinal disorders (g) Colic (h) Diarrhoea (i) Abdominal distension (j) Fevers (k) Heart diseases (l) Cough (m) Nausea/vomiting (n) Nervine (o) Bronchitis (p) Headache (q) Toothache (r) Liver diseases	**Dry–ginger** Shunti fine powder if taken regularly for 40 days gives relief in Rheumatoid Arthritis. It is a good digestive as well. Dose: 3 grams with milk twice a day.

64. Taleesapatri	(a) Asthma/Bronchial diseases (b) Cough (c) Indigestion (d) Consumption (e) Cold (f) Vomiting	**Talisadi churna** It is a very popular ayurvedic powder made from talisapatra etc. It is a proven remedy for respiratory problems like cough, cold, asthma etc. 5 grams of this sweet powder well mixed in a cup of milk should be taken twice a day.
65. Twak	(a) Throat diseases (b) Headache (c) Bladder diseases (d) Vomiting/diarrhoea	It is one of the components of popularly known **'trijataka'** indicated in cough, cold, etc. It is an aromatic, spice added to the food for flavour.
66. Trivrit	(a) Worms (b) Intestinal diseases (c) Fevers (d) Swelling (e) Anaemia (f) Constipation (chronic) (g) Liver diseases (h) Piles (i) Jaundice (j) Visarpa (k) Consumption	—
67. Tuvaraka	(a) Itching (b) Skin diseases/leprosy (c) Worms (d) Bleeding diseases (e) Syphilis (f) Rheumatism	**Skin–oil** Tuvaraka tail obtained from the seeds of Tuvaraka is reputed skin oil used in variety of skin problems like itching, wounds etc.
68. Usheera	(a) Fevers (b) Vomiting (c) Thirst (d) Bleeding diseases (e) Visarpa (f) Burning sensation	**Usheerasavam** is the ready made oral liquid drug useful in variety of female complaints like menstrual excessive bleedings. This should be taken along with

	(g) Rheumatism (h) Gout	other medicines.
69. Vacha	(a) Vomiting (b) Constipation (c) Abdominal distention (d) Colic (e) Urinary diseases (f) Epilepsy (g) Worms/infections (h) Swellings (i) Acidity (children)	**Caution** Vacha is a good drug for epilepsy but it should be used under medical supervision only.
70. Bakuchi	(a) Hair tonic (b) Skin diseases (c) Vomiting (d) Asthma/bleeding diseases (e) Cough (f) Swelling (g) Vitiligo	**Caution** The only drug for (white patches) vitiligo but this has many side effects, like eruption of blisters, burning sensation etc. As such, under medical supervision only it should be tried.
71. Vamsalochana	(a) Cough (b) Urinary diseases (c) Consumption (d) Asthma/Bronchial diseases (e) Dysentery (f) Fever (g) Bleeding diseases (h) Male impotency/ sterility	**Caution** Now a days synthetic variety of vamsalochana is only available. One should avoid it.
72. Vasa	(a) Bleeding diseases (b) Cough (c) Consumption (d) Vomiting (e) Skin disorders (f) Fevers (g) Thirst (h) Asthma/breathing diseases (i) Bronchitis	**Natural cough syrup** Vasa is a versatile green remedy, its applications are many. Vasa leaves juice 2 tsf + tulasi leave juice 1 tsf + betel leaves juice 2 tsf well mixed in 2 tea spoon full of pure honey is the natural cough syrup.

73. **Vibheetaki**	(a) Worms (b) Eye diseases (c) Dysentery/diarrhoea (d) Throat diseases (e) Sore throat (f) Hair loss	**For Blackening of hair** Apply fine powder of this to scalp and hair for half to one hour, weekly once, atleast for 3 months to get encouraging results.
74. **Vidanga**	(a) Worms (b) Colic (c) Intestinal diseases (d) Abdominal distension (e) Headache	**In worms** Powder the dry fruits of embelia ribes (Vidanga), 10gms of powder at bed time on first day followed by 1gm twice a day with hot water for next 10 days is the ideal course on mode.
75. **Vidhari**	(a) Male impotency/ sterility (b) Sore throat (c) Urinary diseases (d) Complexion enhances (e) Bleeding diseases (f) Burning sensation (g) Consumption (h) Diabetes	**Arthritis** Vidari churna is a good supplement for Arthritis patients. 5gms of powder well mixed in a glass of milk twice a day is an ideal application especially in osteo-arthritis (O.A.)
76. **Yashtimadhu**	(a) Eye diseases (b) Complexion (c) Male diseases/ impotency (d) Hair fall (e) Sore throat (f) Bleeding diseases (g) Vomiting (h) Thirst (i) Cosumption (j) Urinary diseases (k) Cough / Cold (l) Asthma (m) Fevers (n) Burning sensation	**Allergy** In chronic Urticaria (Skin Allergy) fine powder of yastimadhu well mixed in ghee should be given twice a day for 15 days. It resolves the burning problem spontaneously. Dose 3gm-5gm with pure ghee twice a day.

5.

Home Herbal Kit for Common Diseases

Every home should have the following safe, simple herbal drugs stock in the form of a kit or box for solving everyday health problems like cough, cold, indigestion, diarrhoea, stomachache, headache etc.

These herbals can be used without any fear of side effects or complications, provided they are identified properly and stored cleanly. These herbal powders/pills must be replaced with fresher ones as these may lose their curing potency on long storage. Minimum quantity of these herbals should be maintained in the house holds, so that they can be discarded on expiry (after six months time) without much loss.

General Instructions

1. Procure these green remedies from a reputed raw drug dealer or Ayurvedic medical store.
2. In case of any doubt regarding the identity of the herb/plant ask the locally available Ayurvedic / Unani doctors, who are well versed with these herbals.
3. As far as possible procure finished product only, as the processing is a difficult work.
4. However in case of leaves like tulasi neem etc. they should be collected fresh from the home gardens or nearby places.
5. Do not collect the herbals/flowers/leaves etc. from any unhygienic areas like grave yards, unwholesome water tanks, surroundings areas of chemical factories etc., as they may get contaminated with unwanted toxins.
6. Before using them wash them properly by soaking in a bucket full of water for 2 –3 hours so that any agrochemical/pesticides left over them is washed away.
7. All these powders should be poured into suitable glass jars, bottles and labeled properly in the known languages.
8. To measure, a steel tea-spoon should be used. Generally 1 tea spoon full means 5 grams of powder or 5 milliliters of liquid. 1 tsp = 15 grams or 15ml.
9. All the green remedies should be consumed along with some hot water when it turns luke warm. This aids in rapid absorption of the drug. However in specified conditions cold water can also be used.

10. Unless specified the doses mentioned are adult doses only. For children, reduced doses are to be used as recommended in each case or as per the advice of the local herbalist/ayurvedic physician.

Green Plants Which can be Grown in One's Compound

1. Neem	Azadirachta indica
2. Malabar Nut Tree (Adulsa)	Adhatoda vasica
3. Pomegranate	Punica granatum
4. Aloe	Aloe barbedensis
5. Tinospora	Tinospora cordifolia
6. Ginger	Zinziber officinalis
7. Holy Basil (Tulsi)	Ocimum sanctum
8. Mint Leap	Mentha spicata
9. Coriander	Coriandrum sativum
10. Curry Leaf	Murraya koeingi
11. Drumstick	Moringa olifera
12. Mango	Mangifera indica
13. Papaya	Carica papaya
14. Basil Leaf	Basilla alba
15. Fenugreek	Triogonella foenum graecum

Constituents and their Applications

Name of the Drug/Herbals

1. Triphala

(Combination in equal proportions of haritaki, vibhitaki & amalaki)

Form : Fine powder / coarse powder for kashaya.

Application

a) **Constipation / piles:** Add 1 to 2 tsf of triphala churna to a cup full of luke warm water and drink before going to bed daily. This ensures clear motions.

b) **Maintenance of eye sight and blackening of hair:** 1 tsf powder well mixed in pure ghee should be consumed orally along with a cup of warm milk, preferably on empty stomach in the early morning.

c) **For blackening of hair:** Mix required quantity of triphala powder with curd or water and apply on the scalp and hairs. Leave it for 30 min to 1 hr. Later wash the hair with plain water.

2. Neem (Azadirachta Indica)

Form : Leaves Powder

Applications

Well dried neem leaves should be powdered, filtered and kept in a clean bottle. Every three months, this powder should be replaced with fresh powder as the efficacy is likely to be affected.

The freshly prepared one can be successfully used in many every day health problems as indicated below :-

1) As external application in skin diseases like itching, eczema and wounds, the powder mixed in pure coconut oil should be applied on the affected areas.

2) As a bath powder, it can be added to a bucket full of hot water (2 tsp).

Internal Uses

1. Neem powder is the drug of choice in many skin problems like eczema, psoriasis, wounds, acne, pimples and abscesses. It is a good antiseptic as well as blood purifier.

   The powder can be encapsulated in the home itself (by filling the powder into empty 500 mg capsules).

2. When there is no medical aid available in the early cases of jaundice and fevers, this neem powder in the form of tea decoction should be given to the patients for immediate arrest of progress of disease. Sugar can be added to the neem decoction if desired.
3. Neem can also be used as dental sticks for regular mouth washing in dental and gum problems.
4. In worm infestations : Tender leaves of neem grinded into paste when taken early morning on empty stomach in a small dose of pea head size relieves all types worm infestations.

In short, neem is a wonderful herbal drug a herbalist cannot ignore.

3. Trikatu

Combination of	1 part Sunthi	:	Dry Ginger
	2 parts Pippali	:	Long Pepper
	3 parts Maricha	:	Black Pepper

From : Fine powder

Application

It is chiefly useful in respiratory problems like:

a) **Common cold and cough** — 3 gms of trikatu fine powder well mixed in a glass of hot milk should be used thrice a day.

For children 1 ½ gm of the powder well mixed in pure honey +1/2 tsf of tulasi juice can be given twice a day.

b) **Indigestion** – It can also be used in loss of appetite as well as in indigestion. It promotes the secretion of digestive juices.

Caution : Persons with acidity problems should not use this as it may aggravate the condition.

4. Ashwagandha Churna (Withania Somnifera)

Popularly known as Indian ginseng

Form : Powder

Applications : It is a versatile herbal that can be used in many complaints. It is a reputed nervine tonic and general tonic.

a) General health promotive : 5 gms of powder well mixed in a glass of milk should be taken once a day preferably at bed time. This helps in many ways and keeps one physically and mentally alert.

b) Joint pains in old age is one of the common problems which is due to a degenerative process, and ashwagandha being a good nutritive tonic, works to prevent further loss of bone tissue. 5 gms of powder well mixed in a cup of warm milk should be taken twice a day for 40 days continuously.

c) Underweight— In underweight people also this helps. 5 gms twice a day well boiled in milk can be used. This is known as ashwagandha Kheerapaka i.e ashwagandha processed in milk.

5. Amla Powder (Indian Gooseberry)

The very fine powder obtained from dried amla fruits duly fortified with amla fresh juice is available as a readymade preparation under the name "Amalaki rasayana" in the ayurvedic medical stores. This is available in 60 gms pack.. One such pack should be placed in the home kit for the following medicinal uses:

1. Acidity – Give ½ tsf powder well mixed in 2tsf of pure honey thrice a day for a sure and sustained relief.
2. Health promotion - In emaciated or run down condition this amla powder, should be given 1 tsf twice a day with a glass of lukewarm milk and sugar. It increases appetite, promotes well being and increases body weight.

Other uses can also be referred in the section of individual drugs appended.

6. Shatavari Powder (Asparagus Racemosus)

This can also be procured from the ayurvedic medical shop and kept in the home chest. 100 grams pack is enough.

Important Uses

1. To increase lactation ; 1 tsf of powder well mixed in a cup of warm milk given twice a day increases mothers milk adequately.
2. To increase weight : 5 gms powder well mixed in milk twice a day.

Further shatavari is a good natural antacid. It can be used by the acidity and ulcer patients regularly. If used in excessive quantity it causes indigestion, therefore one has to use this keeping in view his digestive capacity.

Other uses can be referred to the individual drug section of this book.

7. Bhaskara Lavan

Form : Powder

Readymade preparation should be kept in the home chest. Regular dose is 3gms twice a day with warm water. It is effective in indigestion, gas problems, abdominal pain and decreased appetitie.

8. Chandana

Sandal wood powder is used as a face pack, in pimples, acne and black spots over the face. It is a beauty aid.

9. Haridra Powder (Turmeric)

1. Useful in treating all stones, anti-cancer agent, anti-oxidant.
2. It is used for injuries and skin problems.
3. It can be used as cream or ointment.
4. Used in beauty aid, removes pimples, improves skin quality and discourages unwanted hair on feminine skin.

10. Hingu Powder

Fried hingu powder is highly useful in gas problems, indigestion and abdominal pain. 2gm should be used with warm water twice a day.

11. Shunti Powder (Dry Ginger Powder)

It is good for arthritis, indigestion, cold and prevents travel sickness. (Refer section on individual drugs for further details.)

Green Remedies Used as Anti-diabetics

S. No.	Hindi Name	Botanical Name	Ayurvedic Name	Availability	Parts Used	Chemical Composition
1.	(Neem) Neem	Azadirachta indica	Nimba	Throughout India	Leaves & oil Azadisone	Nimbin, Nimbosterol, Azadisone
2.	(Jamun) Jambo	Syzygium cumini	Jambo	Throughout India	Leaves & seeds	Beta-pinene, Limoriene Beta-sitosterol
3.	(Gurmar) Periploca	Gymnema sylvestris	Mesha shringi	Central India	Leaf	G.acid and Glycoside
4.	(Karela) Bitter Gourd	Momordica charantia	Karavellaka	Throughout India	Fruits pulp, leaves	Momordicin, Charantine & Phenolics A crystalline product named p-insulin
5.	(Vijsar) Malabar Kind Tree	Pterocarpus marsupium	Beejaka	Throughout India	Heartwood	Terpenoids, Tannins, Pterosupin Glycosides, Flavoures Beta-sitosterol
6.	(Kuth) Kuth	Sausseurea lappa	Kushtha	Kashmir, Himachal pradesh, Garhwal	Root	Kushthin, Sitosterol
7.	(Guduchi) Tinospora	Tinospora cordifolia	Guduchi	All over India	Stem, Whole plant	Tinosporine, Giloin & Hepatocosa
8.	(Methi) Fenugreek	Papilonacaea methi	Methika	All over India	Seeds & Leaves	Essential oil 6% calcium, phosphorous & protein etc.

Green Remedies Helpful in Cancer

VEGETABLES/PLANTS/FRUITS	
Vegetables	
Cauliflower Cabbage Garlic Tomatoes Onions Turmeric	**REMARKS** : These possess some sulphur containing compounds which are anti-cancer agents.
Plants	
Banafsa: *(viola odorata)* Sadabahar: *(catharanthus roseus)* Tea: *(camellia sinensis)* Til: *(sesamum indicum)* Shahjan: *(Drumstick)*	
Fruits	
Anannas Sharifa Amla Barhal	

*Curcumin, a yellow pigment in turmeric is found to be non-steroidal and is an anti-cancer agent.

General Tonics

Immunity Boosters

Ayurveda and other eastern systems of medicine offer an excellent range of immunity enhancers, which can be easily grown or procured in both rural as well as urban settings.

1. **Shatavari** : Botanically known as Asparagus racemosus, it is one of the best and safe immunity boosters and a good strength promoter. Though it is equally useful in both the sexes, its use in females is more suitable.

   Wash tubers of shatavari, remove outer skin layer and crush well, then collect extracted juice. Mix about ½ cup of this fresh juice in ½ cup of pure milk add 1tsp of sugar and boil on gentle fire for 5 minutes.

2. **Ashwagandha** : Botanically known as Withania somnifera is a globally recognized tonic. It is called as Indian ginseng. It is a good nervine and general tonic indicated in rundown conditions. Its regular use boosts up the body immunity and resistance power.

   Prepare decoction with roots of ashwagandha in good and clean vessel. Take ½ a cup twice a day for 7 – 21 days.

3. **Guduchi** : Botanically well known as Tinospora cordifolia, is an ever green herb which spreads over trees especially on neem trees, useful in a variety of diseases in addition to its immunity promoting quality.

   Prepare decoction with stem of guduchi, consume orally ½ a cup decoction twice a day for 40 days. 1 tsp of pure honey can be added if one desires.

4. **Vidari** : Botanically known as Ipomoea mouritiana , is a good strengthening drug and adds bulk to the body.

   Prepare decoction with tubers of vidari and take ½ a cup in the morning and evening with a cup of milk for 40 days.

5. **Amlaki** : Fresh fruits, popularly known as Emblica officinalis, is an ever green remedy and tonic. Regular use of this promotes health and strength. During the season, 2 – 3 fresh amlaki fruits should be crushed to extract the juice. This juice can be taken twice a day well mixed in a spoon full of honey.

   For those people who smoke and chew pan, daily intake of amlaki juice prevents acidity, heart burn and constipation apart from improving appetite and complexion.

Memory Boosters

There are many green herbs /plants which are grown around us in our compounds/ or open spaces, which are highly useful in loss of memory, concentration and sleep.

Some of such most common green remedies are listed with necessary instructions :-

1. **Mandukaparni**- Botanically known as Centella asiatica, it is the common memory booster, especially for school-going children.

   Prepare milk decoction with whole plant of Centella asciatica. Take a cup at bed time daily for 40 days for positive results.

   For children ½ a cup should be given before going to bed.

2. **Brahmi** : An equally effective plant, it is botanically known as Bacopa monnieri. It's fresh leaves juice in the dosage of 15ml to 30ml with some honey is generally taken at bed time for 40 days for sustained results. However diabetic patients are instructed not to mix honey; instead, only juice should be taken. Other brain tonics available in one's home are : Pure ghee & milk, good reading habits, dhyana or concentration, avoidance of green or red chillies, strong spices & excessive volume in music are essential to gain memory power.

Liver Correctives (Tonics) and Appetizers

1. Fresh and green ginger is the best appetizer easily available in everyone's home.

   Take some fresh ginger and cut into small pieces, add little bit of salt or sugar, mix well and chew ½ hour before mealtime. It is a very good appetizer and digestive and relieves gas formation after meals.

   People with high blood pressure should not add salt, instead sugar can be added; similarly diabetics should not add sugar.

2. Haritaki or harad botanically well known as Terminalia chebula is a proven liver tonic and laxative. Crush some dried fruit bark of harad and make fine powder. 1 tsp powder well mixed in a cup of luke warm water should be consumed at bed time for 40 days.

3. Prepare decoction with stem of guduchi (Tinopora cordifolia). 1 cup of this decoction should be consumed at bed time regularly by alcoholics for liver protection.

4. Crush leaf pulp of kumari popularly known as Aloe barbadensis, 2 tsp of juice twice a day, keeps the liver in good form.

   Avoidance of fatty food, fried food is must. Fresh vegetables and fruits are highly useful.

Breast Milk Enhancers

Mother's milk is the best food for infants. No other costly baby food can substitute it. Therefore Ayurveda offers certain specific herbs which can increase the flow of milk to a certain extent. These are known as galactogogues.

However, before taking these herbs a full medical check-up is required to rule out any constitutional disorders.

1. **Shatavari** - Botanically known as Asparagus racemosus, it is the herb of choice. Fresh juice of tubers or powder of dried tubers is generally used.

   Dose : fresh juice 20 ml added to a cup of milk , twice a day.

   Powder : 5 gms added to a cup of milk + sugar, twice a day.

   Now-a-days to make it more acceptable to modern mothers, sugar coated granules are marketed under different brand names like shatavarex etc. 5 gms of granules added to a glass of milk twice a day is the recommended dosage.

   Further shatavari is a good appetite stimulant, brain stimulant, aphrodisiac and above all it is a rich nutritive tonic. Being a natural anti-acid it does not cause side effects like constipation or diarrhoea. It normalizes the gastric pH and has longer duration of action.

2. **Vidari Kanda** – Botanically popular as Ipomea maurtiana, it is another effective herbal drug for increasing the breast milk.

   Decoction of dried tubers is prepared and taken in the dosage schedule of 30ml twice a day. Sugar can be mixed in the decoction. This should be taken for 7 days; after a short gap if required the same can be repeated.

   Apart from these two herbals, there is an exclusive group of herbal drugs known as stanya janana i.e galactogogue drugs described in ayurvedic system of medicine.

Note : Depending on the availability of the herbals any one of the herbs can be used.

Mother and Child Care

Green Remedy	Useful Condition	Market Preparation
I. During Pregnancy		
(Anar) Pomegranate	morning sickness nausea, loss of appetite or poor appetite, anaemia, diarrhoea, stomachache	**Anardana Churna** 1 tsp twice (Dabur) Dadimadi Lehya 1tsp twice (Sandu)
(Giloy) Tinospora	fever, body-pains, thirst, for general health promotion	**Guduchi Satv** (Baidyanath) 1/2 tsp honey twice a day
(Khas) Usheera	bad body odour, burning sensation, over sweating	**Usheerasava** 15 ml twice a day (Sandu)
(Kamal) Lotus	burning sensation, excessive sweating, thirst	**Usheerasava** 15 ml twice a day
Shatavari	burning urine, general weakness, difficulty in urination, general tonic	**Shatavarex** granules 5gms twice a day with milk (Zandu)
(Amla) Indian Gooseberry	as a routine general tonic	**Chywanprasha** (Zandu) 1 tsp twice daily
Brahmi	spasm, epilepsy, memory loss	**Vita** granules (DAP) 1 tsp with milk twice a day
(Punarnava) Hogweed	anaemia, swelling over the body, giddiness, urinary obstruction	**Punarnavasav** (Sandu) 15 ml twice a day
(Bilai Kand) kudzu Indian	under weight, general weakness, fever, cold	**Vidari Churna** 5gms twice a day with milk
(Elaichi) Cardamom	vomiting, morning sickness, skin eruptions, execessive watering in the mouth.	**Eladi Pills** (Dabur) 1 tab thrice a day to be chewed

(Asgandha) Ashwagandha	swelling, vertigo, general health tonic, joints pains	**Stressnil Caps** (Baidyanath) 1 tab thrice a day
(Adrak & Sont) Wet & dry Ginger	indigestion, cold, stomach upsets, constipation, poor appetite, increased appetite	**Nagaradi Vati** (Baidyanath) 1 tab thrice a day
(Gokharu) Puncture-vine	blood in urine, burning urine, swellings	**Gokshuradi Kada** (Sandu) 15 ml thrice a day
(Ajowan) Ajwoin	indigestion, fever, abdominal pain, gas problem	**Ajamoda Arka** (Impcops) 1tsp thrice a day
(Musali Kand) Musli	prevents threatened abortions and general tonic for pregnant women	**Musaliark** (Baidyanath) 1 tsp twice a day
(Mulhati) Liquorice	acidity, burning sensation, throat irritations, cough	**Yasti Madhu Churna** (Zandu) 3 gms twice a day with milk
(Bel) Bel Fruit	diarrhoea, dysentry, abdominal pain, amoebiasis	**Antisar Capsules** (Chandrika) 1 cap twice a day
(Angur) Raisins	giddiness, thirst, anemia, nutritive & cooling	**Drakshadi Lehya** (Dabur) 1 tsp twice a day

II. During Lactation

Shatavari	Purifies breast milk, makes it more digestible, promotes lactation	**Shatavarex Granules** 1 tsp twice daily with milk
Ashwagandha	-do-	**Stress Com** (Dabur)
(Bilal Kand) Indian Kudzu	-do-	**Vidari Kalpa**
Angur	keeps up mother's health	**Angurasav** (Dabur)

III. Child Care & Pediatric Problems		
(Amla) Gooseberry	cold, cough, constipation, mouth ulcers, underweight, a health tonic	**Chywanprash** (Dabur) 1 tsp twice a day with a cup of warm milk
Brahmi	spasmodic pains, epileptic fits, poor or loss of memory, brain tonic	**Braḥmi Vati** (Dabur) 1 tab twice a day
(Kalamegh) Chirayata, Chiretta	malarial and other fevers, cold etc.	Antimal tabs (Bajaj) 1 tab thrice a day with hot water
(Musta) Nutgrass	vommiting, diarrhoea, stomach ache, pediatric tonic	**Mustakarishta** (Dabur) 15 ml twice a day
(Ajmud) Ajowan	digestion problems	**Ajamoda Arka** (Baidyanath) 10ml twice a day with luke warm water
(Atis) Atis Root	fever, diarrhoea, vomiting in children	**Samshamana Vati** (Baidyanath) 1 tab twice a day
(Gorbach) Sweet Flag	memory and mental ill health, improves intelligence	**Memorin Cap** (Phyto pharma) 1 cap daily with milk
(Bel) Fruit	intestinal problems like dystentery, pain etc	**Bilwadi Lehya** (Sandu) 1 tsp twice daily
(Mulahati) Liqudrice	cough, throat problems	**Yashti Tabs** (Impcops) 1 tab twice a day
(Angur) Raising	vertigo, constipation, anaemia, general health tonic	**Draksharishta** (Baidyanath) 15 ml twice a day

Dosage for Children

Age in Months	Fresh Juice Dose (Swarasa)	Decoction Dose (Kwatha)
Upto 1 month	0.25 ml	0.50 ml
Upto 2 months	0.50 ml	1.00 ml
Upto 3 months	0.75 ml	1.50 ml
Upto 4 months	1.00 ml	2.00 ml
Upto 5 months	1.25 ml	2.50 ml
Upto 6 months	1.50 ml	3.00 ml
Above 6 months to 1 yr	3.00 ml	6.00 ml
Upto 2 years	5 ml	10 ml
Upto 3 years	7 ml	14 ml
Upto 4 years	9 ml	18 ml
Upto 5 years	10 ml	21 ml
Upto 6 years	13 ml	26 ml
Upto 10 years	21 ml	42 ml
Upto 16 years	34 ml	68 ml
Above 16 to 70 years	34 ml	68 ml

Instructions on How to Select a Remedy for a Particular Health Complaint

1. To find out which herb or herbs are recommended for a particular health complaint or disease. First refer to the "disease wise green remedies" index and then refer that particular herb in the green remedies description section.
2. Self-diagnosis is not advisable. Consult an ayurvedic physician or herbalist to ascertain the nature of the health problem.
3. The dosages mentioned are applicable to adults only. For children and old age people, the dosage has to be cut down to ½ of the adult dose or as advised by physician.

Glossary of Medical Terms

Abscess : A localised collection of pus caused by suppuration in a tissue

Acne : A term denoting an inflammatory disease occurring in or around the sebaceous glands

Acrid : Biting, pungent

Albuminuria : The presence of serum albumin and serum globulin in the urine

Alexipharmic : Antidote to poison

Alexiteric : Protective to infectious diseases

Alopecia : Loss of hair – a malady in which the hair falls from one or more circumscribed round or oval areas, leaving the skin smooth and white

Alterative : Causing a favourable change in the disordered functions of the body or metabolism

Amenorrhoea : Failure of menstruation

Amentia : An arrest of the development of the mind from birth to early age

Anaemia : Lack of enough blood causing paleness

Analgesic : An anodyne, a pain killer

Anaphrodisiac : Having the power to lessen or inhibit sexual feeling

Anasarca : Diffused dropsy in the skin and subcutaneous tissue

Anorexia : A condition of having lost the appetite for food.

Anthelmintic : Destroying or expelling worms.

Antidote : An agent which neutralises or opposes the action of a poison

Antiemetic : An agent that relieves vomiting

Antiperiodic : Preventing the regular recurrence of a disease

Antipruritic : Preventing or relieving itching

Antipyretic : Counteracting fever

Antiscorbutic : Acting against scurvy

Antiseptic : A chemical sterilising substance to kill or control pathogenic microbes

Antispasmodic : Opposing spasms or convulsions

Anuria : Complete cessation of the secretion and excretion of urine

Aperient : A laxative or mild cathartic

Aphrodisiac : A drug which stimulates sexual desire

Arthralgia : Pain in a joint

Arthritis : Inflammation of a joint

Atrophy : Wasting of a tissue or organ

Balanitis : A condition of inflammation of the glans penis or of the glans of clitoris

Beriberi : A deficiency disease caused by imbalance of carbohydrate and Vitamin B

Cachexia : Depressed habit of mind

Calculus : A concretion formed in any part of the body usually compounds of salts of organic or inorganic acids

Carbuncle : An infection of the skin and subcutaneous tissue by Staphylococcus aureus.

Cardiopathy : A morbid condition of the heart

Carminative : Drug curing flatulence

Cataract : Opacity in the crystalline lens of the eye which may be partial or complete

Catarrh : Inflammation of a mucous membrane, usually associated with an increase in the amount of normal secretion of mucus.

Cathartic : Having the power of cleansing the bowels – purgative

Cephalic : A remedy for disorders of the head.

Cerebropathy : Any disorder of the brain.

Cholera : A severe infectious epidemic disease due to Vibrio cholerae

Cirrhosis : A general term meaning progressive fibrous tissue overgrowth in an organ

Colic : A severe spasmodic griping pain

Colitis : Inflammation of the colon

Collyrium : An eye-salve or eye-wash

Coma : The state of complete loss of consciousness

Conjunctivitis : Inflammation of the conjunctiva

Consumption : Pulmonary tuberculosis

Contraceptive : Any agent or device used to prevent conception

Convulsion : A violent involuntary contraction of the skeletal musculature.

Corn : A small circumscribed painful horny growth.

Cystitis : Inflammation of a bladder, especially the urinary bladder

Dandruff : Dead scarf-skin separating in small scales and entangled in the hair

Demulcent : Soothing

Dental caries : Decay of teeth

Deodorant : Removing the odour

Depurative : An agent that purifies blood

Diaphoresis : Sweating

Diaphoretic : A drug which induces perspiration

Diphtheria : A specific infectious disease caused by virulent strains of a bacillus

Disinfectant : Having a lethal effect upon germs

Diuretic : Promoting the flow of urine.

Dizziness : Any sensation of imbalance of a stable relationship with the immediate environment.

Dropsy : An excessive accumulation of clear or watery fluid in any of the tissues or cavities of the body

Dysmenorrhoea : Difficult or painful menstruation

Dyspnoea : Difficulty in breathing

Dyspepsia : Indigestion

Dystocia : Difficult parturition (birth).

Dysuria : Difficulty or pain while passing urine

Eclampsia : An attack of convulsion associated with hypertension in pregnancy

Eczema : A non-contagious inflammatory disease of the skin with much itching and burning

Elephantiasis : Gross lymphatic oedema of the limbs leading to hypertrophy

Emetic : Causing vomiting

Emmenagogue : Medicine intended to restore the menses (menstrual flow).

Emphysema : A pathologic accumulation of air in tissues or organs

Empyema : Accumulation of pus in a body cavity

Encephalitis : Inflammation of the brain and spinal cord due to infection.

Encephalopathy	: Any degenerative brain disease
Enuresis	: Involuntary voiding of urine
Epilepsy	: An affection of the nervous system resulting from excessive or disordered discharge of cerebral neurons.
Epistaxis	: Bleeding from the nose
Erysipelas	: An inflammatory disease generally affecting the face marked by a bright redness of the skin.
Expectorant	: Aiding the secretion of the mucous membrane of the air passages and the removal of fluid by spitting.
Febrifuge	: Anything which reduces fever
Filariasis	: Infection with filarial nematode worms.
Fistula in ano	: An open channel from the anus or rectum to the skin near the anus.
Flatulence	: Presence of excessive gas in the stomach or intestine.
Galactagogue	: Medicine that promotes secretion of milk
Galactorrhoea	: Excessive or spontaneous flow of milk.
Gangrene	: Necrosis and putrefaction of tissue due to lack of blood supply
Gastroenteritis	: Inflammation of the mucous coat of the stomach and intestine due to bacterial infection.
Germicidal	: Causing destruction of micro-organisms
Gingivitis	: Inflammation of the gingival margins around the teeth accompanied by welling and bleeding.
Glycosuria	: Excretion of sugar in the urine.
Goitre	: Enlargement of the thyroid gland.
Gonorrhoea	: An inflammatory disease of the genitourinary passages characterised by pain and discharge
Haematemesis	: Vomiting of blood
Haematuria	: The presence of blood in the urine
Haemoptysis	: Spitting of blood
Haemorrhoid	: A bleeding pile
Haemostatic	: Styptic
Halitosis	: Offensive odour of the breath
Helminthiasis	: Morbid state due to infestation with worms

Hematorrhoea : Copious haemorrhage

Hemicrania : Headache confined to one side

Hemiplegia : Paralysis of one side of the body

Hepatitis (viral) : Inflammation of the liver; Jaundice

Hepatomegaly : Enlargement of the liver

Hernia : The protrusion of an internal organ through a defect in the wall of the anatomical cavity in which it lies.

Herpes : Inflammation of the skin or mucous membrane with clusters of deep seated vesicles.

Hydrocele : A circumscribed collection of fluid in the tunica vaginalis testis

Hydrophobia : Exaggerated fear of water as in rabies.

Hypertension : High arterial blood pressure

Hyperthermia : A very high body temperature

Hypotension : A fall in blood pressure below the normal level

Hypothermia : Greatly decreased temperature

Hysteria : A neurotic disorder with varying symptoms

Impetigo : An inflammation of the skin associated with discrete vesicles due to streptococcal infection

Impotence : Inability to perform the sexual act due to failure of the reflex mechanism

Insanity : Mental disease of a grave kind

Insomnia : The condition of being unable to sleep

Intoxication : General condition which results following the absorption and diffusion in the body of a soluble poison.

Laryngitis : Inflammation of the larynx.

Laxative : Having the action of loosening the bowel.

Leucoderma : Any white area on the skin

Leucorrhoea : An abnormal mucous discharge from the vagina

Leukaemia : Blood cancer

Lumbago : Pain in mid or lower back

Malignanat : Threatening life or tending to cause death

Melancholia : A mental illness in which the predominant symptom is melancholy, depression of spirits, unhappiness and misery

Menorrhagia : Excessive or prolonged menstruation

Metrorrhagia : Uterine bleeding, usually of normal amount occurring at completely irregular intervals, the period of flow sometimes being prolonged.

Micturition : The act of passing urine

Migraine : A periodic condition with localised headaches, frequently associated with vomiting and sensory disturbances.

Morbid : Belonging or relating to disease

Mumps : Epidemic parotitis, an acute infectious disease caused by a virus

Myalgia : Muscular pain

Mydriasis : Dilatation of the pupil

Narcotic : A drug that induces sleep

Nephritis : Inflammation of the kidneys

Neuralgia : A painful affection of the nerves due to functional disturbances or neuritis.

Notalgia : Pain in the back

Obesity : An excessive accumulation of fat in the body

Odontalgia : Toothache

Opacity : An opaque or non-transparent area

Orchitis : Inflammation of the testis characterised by hypertrophy and pain

Otalgia : Pain in the ear

Pancreatitis : Inflammation of the pancreas

Paraplegia : Stroke affecting one side

Parkinsonism : Parkinson's disease – a disease chracterised by rigidity of muscles and tremor of the hands.

Pectoral : Effective in diseases of the chest

Pertussis : Whooping cough

Pharyngitis : Inflammation of the mucous membrane and underlying part of the pharynx

Phthisis : Any wasting disease in which the whole body or part of the body is involved.

Pneumonia : A general disease in which the essential lesion is an inflammation of the spongy tissue of the lung with consolidation of the alveolar exudate.

Pneumonitis : Inflammation of lung tissue

Poliomyelitis : An acute inflammation of the anterior horn cells of the spinal cord due to an enterovirus infection

Poultice : A soft mush prepared by various substances with oily or watery fluids.

Proctitis : Inflammation of the rectum

Prophylactic : Pertaining to the prevention of the development of a disease

Prurigo : An eruption of the skin causing severe itching.

Pruritis : Itching

Psoriasis : A condition characterised by the eruption of circumscribed discrete and confluent reddish, silvery scaled lesions.

Pyrexia : A condition characterised by the presence of pus

Pyorrhoea : A discharge of pus

Rachilagia : Pain in the vertebral column

Refrigerant : Cooling

Renal calculi : Calculi relating to kidney

Retinitis : Inflammation of the retina

Rheumatalgia : Rheumatic pain

Rhinitis : Inflammation of the nasal mucous membrane.

Rickets : A disturbance of the calcium/phosphorus metabolism which occurs in the growing child as a result of vitamin D deficiency

Roborant : A strengthening agent

Scabies : Sarcoptic infestation of the human skin particularly a contagious skin disease caused by invasion of the epidermis

Scald : The lesion caused by contact with a hot liquid or vapour

Scleritis : Inflammation of the sclera

Scrofula : Tuberculous cervical adenitis with or without ulceration

Scurvy : A deficiency disease due to lack of Vitamin C

Sialogogue : An agent that increases the flow of saliva

Synovitis : Inflammation of the synovial membrane of a joint

Sinusitis : Inflammation affecting the mural epithelium of a sinus

Splenomegaly : Enlargement of the spleen

Stomatitis : Generalised inflammation of the oral mucosa

Styptic : Having the power to arrest bleeding

Suppurative : Pus forming

Syphilis : A contagious venereal disease

Tetanus : An infective disease due to the toxins of Clostridium tetani

Tonsilitis : Inflammation of the tonsil

Toxaemia : The condition of general poisoning caused by the entrance of soluble bacterial toxins into the blood

Trauma : A pathological alteration of the supporting tissues of a tooth due to abnormal occlusion

Trichogenous : Stimulating the growth of hair

Ureteritis : Inflammation of the ureter

Urethritis : Inflammation of the urethra

Urethrorrhea : Abnormal discharge from the urethra

Urolithiasis : Urinary calculi

Urticaria : Nettle rash

Uteritis : Inflammation of the uterus

Vaginitis : Inflammation of the vagina

Vermifuge : A drug that expels worms

Verminosis : Helminthiasis

Vertigo : Dizziness

Wart : A circumscribed cutaneous excrescence

References

1. *"One Hundred useful Drugs"* Edited by Dr. A. Lakshmipathi, Arogya Ashram, Madras

2. *"Adarsh Nighantu"* — Bapalal Vaidya, Chowkhamba Publications

3. *"Bhavprakasha Nighantu"* — Chowkhamba Publications

4. *"Indian Medicinal Plants"* Vol. 1 to 5 , Orient Longman, Arya Vaidya Sala

5. *"Medicinal Plants"* — S. K. Jain

6. *"Spices and Condiments"* — J. S. Pruthi

7. *"Fruits" Ranjit Singh,* Govt. of India Publications.

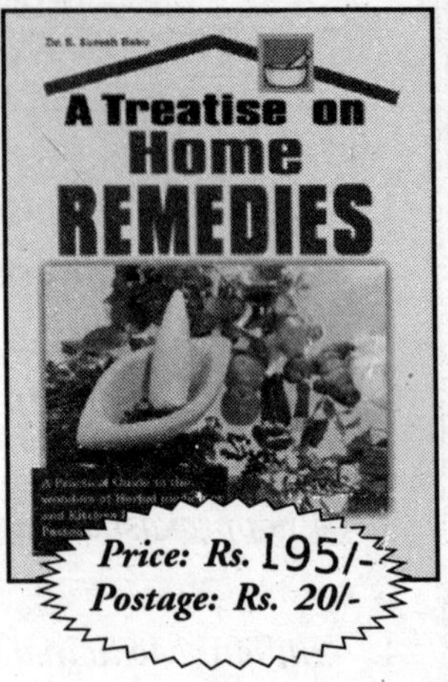

A Treatise on **Home Remedies**

—Dr. S. Suresh Babu, M.D. (Ayur)

Modern medical science may be effective in treating a variety of diseases, but often fails when it comes to chronic problems like gastric-disorders, common cold, respiratory ailments and many others. Here the positive role of traditional, ayurvedic and herbal and home medicines has been proven beyond doubt. This volume brings you an overview of specific problems—backed by not only ayurvedic remedies but also home remedies, along with dietary restrictions and do's & don'ts. From flatulence, constipation, cirrhosis of liver to hepatitis, jaundice and common cold—it covers a broad range. For instance, how a peptic ulcer is formed, and how cold milk is useful in providing relief. Or what are the problems accompanying dysentery and how the 'Bel' fruit is effective in its treatment. The unique feature of the book is the treatment through Home Remedies—items which we've always had at hand in our kitchen like haldi, methi, coconut, cumin (jeera), clove, castor etc. What's more—additional treatments in the form of medicated massages, Hydrotherapy through fomentation methods and Home Beauty aids also bring you useful tips for a healthy and happy life.

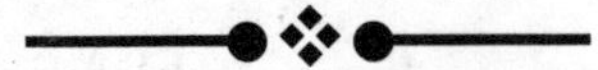

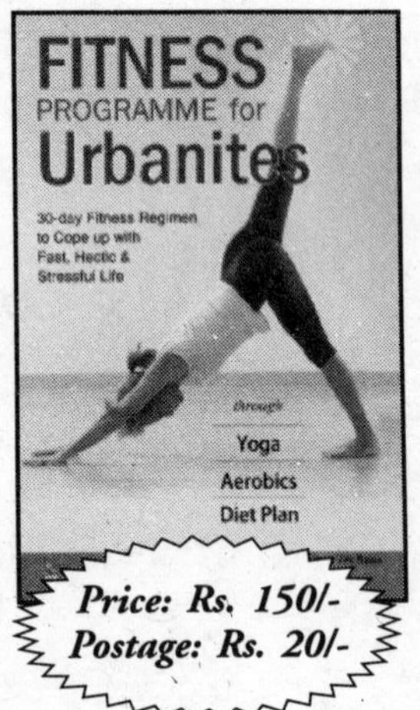

Fitness Programme For Urbanites

—Meghna Virk Bains

FITNESS PROGRAMME for Urbanites, an intensive 30-day fitness regimen, the book has been custom-made to blend with everyone's preference of exercise regimes. The regime that starts at home is for those who prefer the comfort and familiarity of their own surroundings. Aerobics for those who prefer company while they workout. Swimming for those who wish to combine the benefits of a workout with some fun and fluidity. Gyming for those who enjoy the rigorous workout and like to sweat it out. Finally, yoga for those who prefer not just working on their body but also the mind and the soul. The aim is to help you make the ultimate choice, by learning which of the above fitness activities, used singularly or combined, gives you maximum results. In addition, it gives an in-depth understanding of the importance of working out well, eating and sleeping well, and all the other aspects that make for a truly holistic fitness package. The book, therefore, comprehensively works towards transformation of one's lifestyle.

You are What you Eat

It's about how your body responds physically, mentally & spiritually to your food habits

—Tanushree Podder

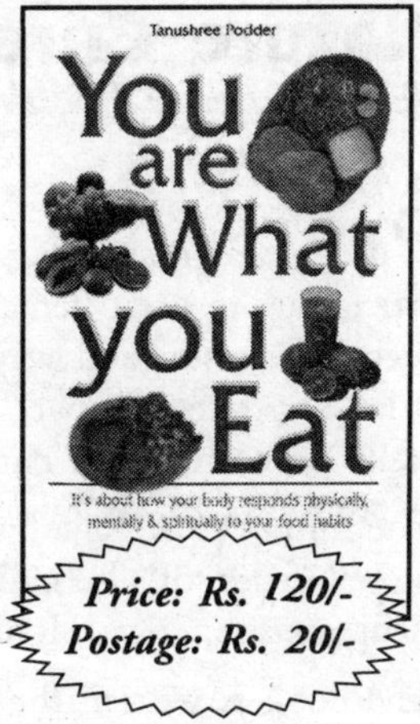

Did you know that food could heal, cure, elevate moods, improve memory, make the brain sharper, provide us with potent energy and fill us with vigour?

Food has been discovered to be the greatest natural pharmacy that is available to human beings. The right food can help us perform to our peak capacity while the wrong food can lead us towards disease and ill health.

The ordinary cabbage and cauliflower could ward off the possibility of cancer, tomatoes can effectively take care of free radicals in today's environment and carrots can provide you with the essential beta-carotene to fight off many diseases. It is surprising how effectively food can alleviate most of our common ailments.

The mysteries of the power of food and the secrets of food elements have been unravelled so that you can use food for other benefits rather than just appeasing hunger.

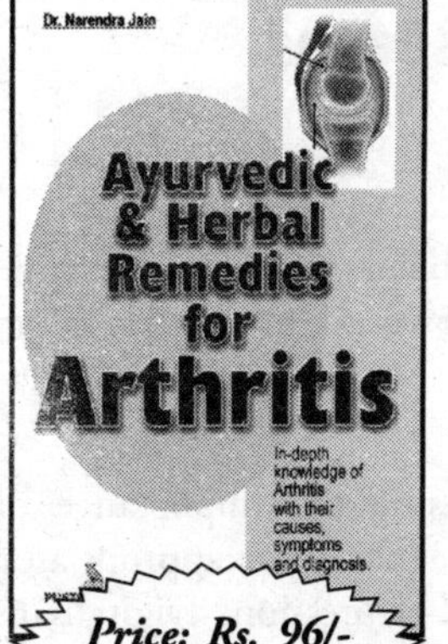

Ayurvedic & Herbal Remedies for Arthritis

—Dr. Narendra Jain

The book, Ayurvedic and Herbal Remedies for Arthritis provides an in-depth knowledge of Arthritis with their causes, symptoms and diagnoses. It primarily focuses on the use of Ayurvedic and Herbal medicines in the treatment of Arthritis and allied conditions. The important aspect of this book is that it takes care to give a detailed description of the herbs available in India and outside India. Hence, the readers from all over the world will find this book interesting and valuable in curing the problems of Arthritis and allied conditions.

More than 35 herbs are mentioned in this book on the basis of their therapeutic value. Monograph of the plants are also given so that the common man can identify them easily. The uniqueness of this book is its special reference on Yoga asanas (with illustrations), Allopathic drugs and pathological tests that are used in the treatment of Arthritis.

Nature Cure at Home

Towards Better Health

—Dr. Rajeshwari

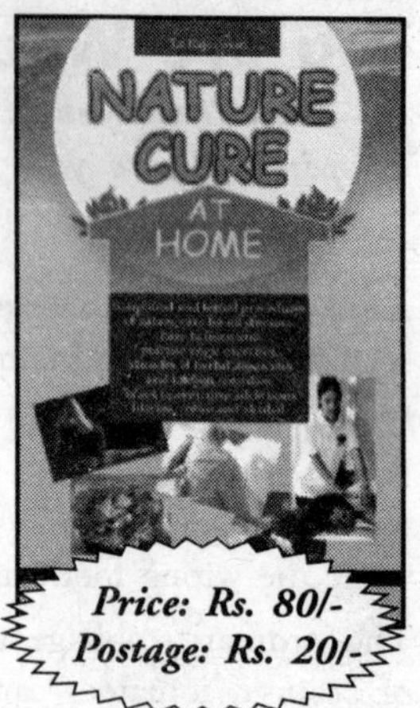

Price: Rs. 80/-
Postage: Rs. 20/-

Public awareness of health is increasing by the day. Health guides and articles are in great demand as people are eager to learn about diseases, their prevention and ways of staying fit, without seeking any medical help. This quest, in part, is due to the realisation that diseases are more easily prevented than cured. This is an encouraging trend.

The author, Dr. Rajeshwari has an illustrious record of practising in several fields of alternative medicines like Naturopathy, Acupressure, Acupuncture, Yoga, Homeopathy and Magnetotherapy.

The book is written for those readers who would like to take care of their own health, using simple remedies, exercises and dietary measures, without exposing themselves to the dangerous side-effects and reactions of potent drugs.

It explains: ❖ Simplified yet effective procedures of nature cure ❖ Herbal remedies for effective treatment of diseases ❖ Curative powers of water.

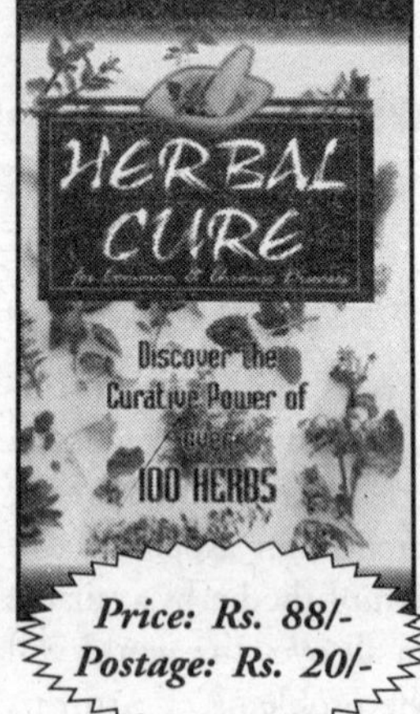

Price: Rs. 88/-
Postage: Rs. 20/-

HERBAL CURE

For Common & Chronic Diseases

—Dr. Syed Aziz Ahmad &
Dr. Shiv Charan Sharma

Traditional herbal remedies have always been valued since time immemorial. Herbal remedies have been known to cure everything, right from spasm to heart diseases and that too without any post-medication blues.

Modern medicine, in fact, is now fast realising the importance of Grandma's cure, which is why herb Rauwolfia has been appropriated by Allopathy to treat high blood pressure and depression, Digitalis to contain the fallouts of heart failure, Cinchona to counter malaria or Neem extracts for diabetes.

In **Herbal Cure** the authors outline the healing and curative properties of more than 100 medicinal plants which are easily available all over the country.

The best part of the book is that in many cases the patients will be able to bring their problems in effective control through simple, readily available herbal solutions.

It also gives information on: ❖ Plant drugs prepared by allopathic drug companies ❖ Plant foods and their nutritive values ❖ Herbal tips to heal and avoid common ailments

More Books on Heath

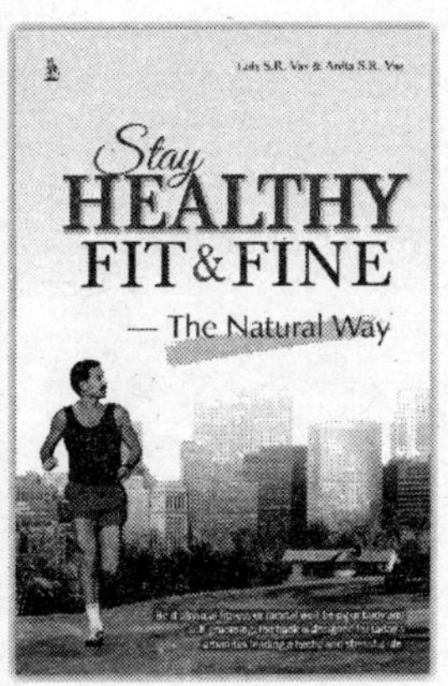

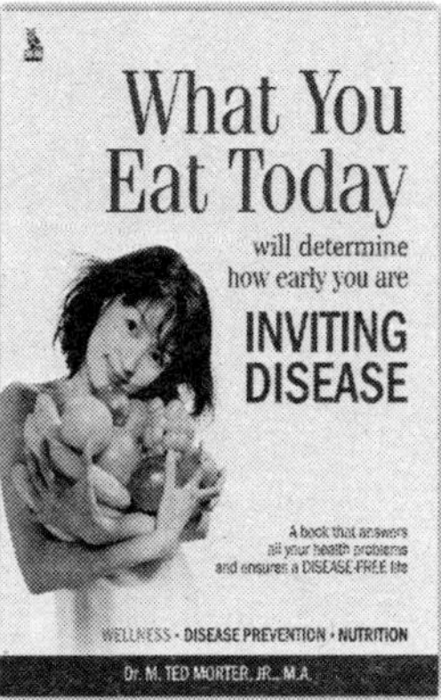

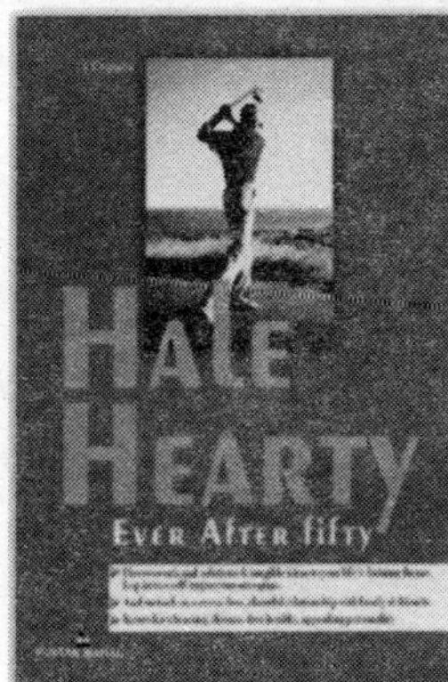

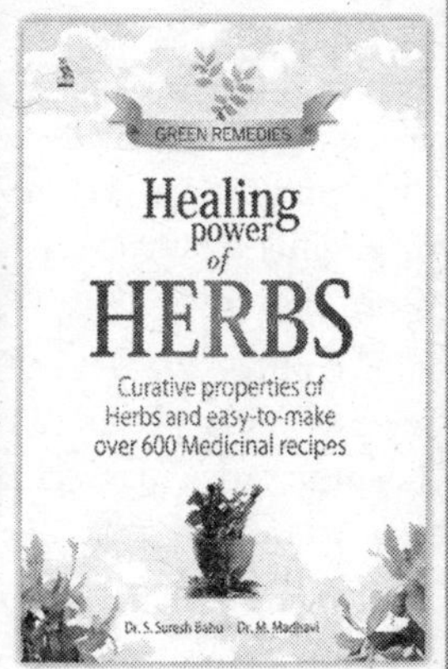

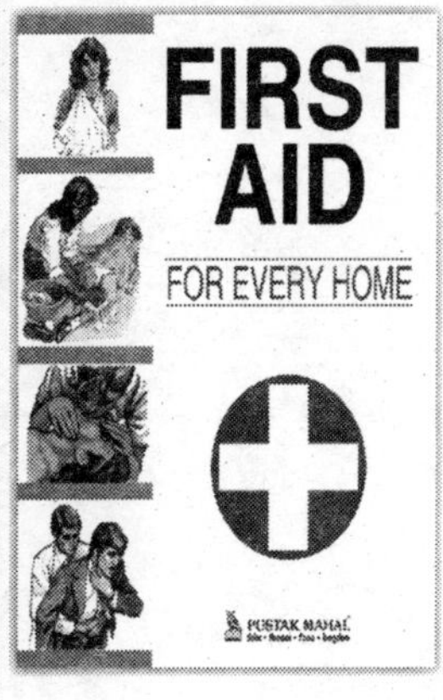

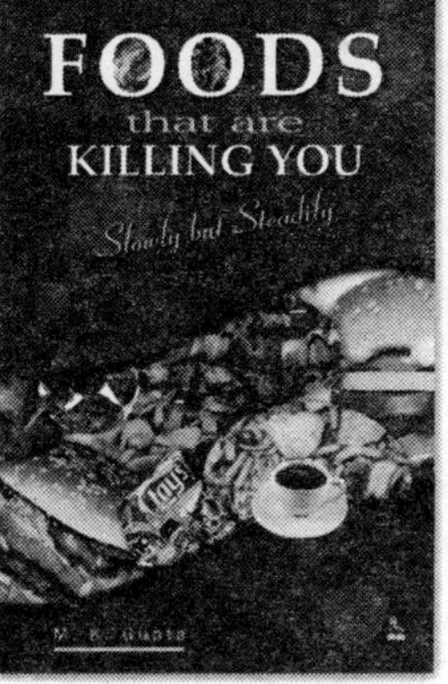

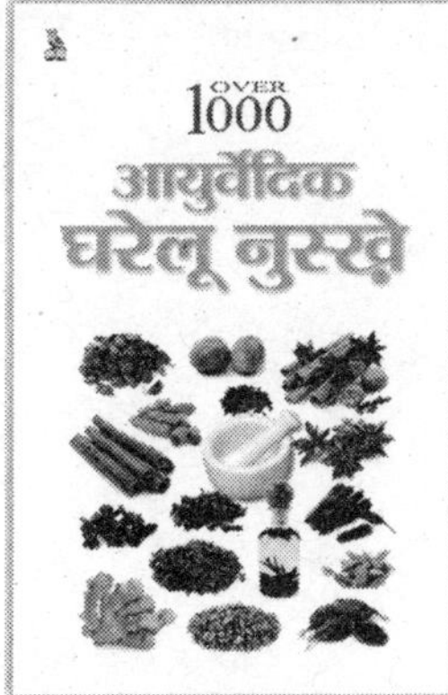

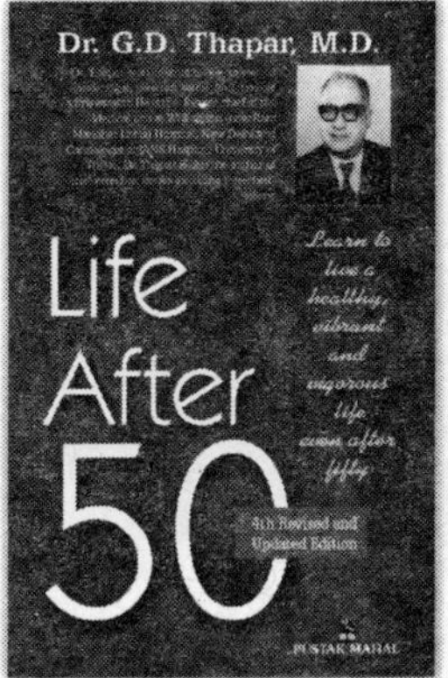

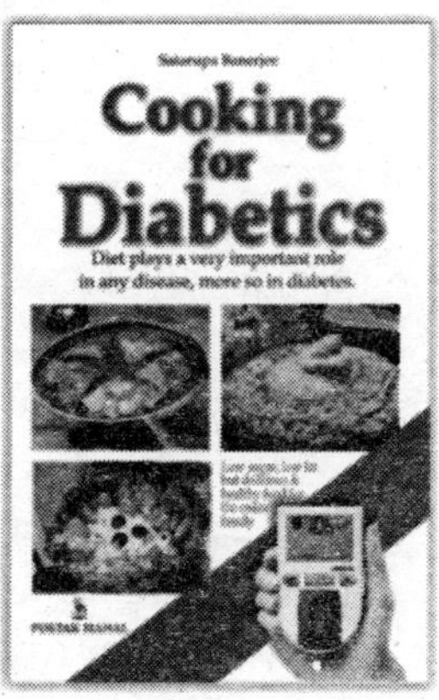

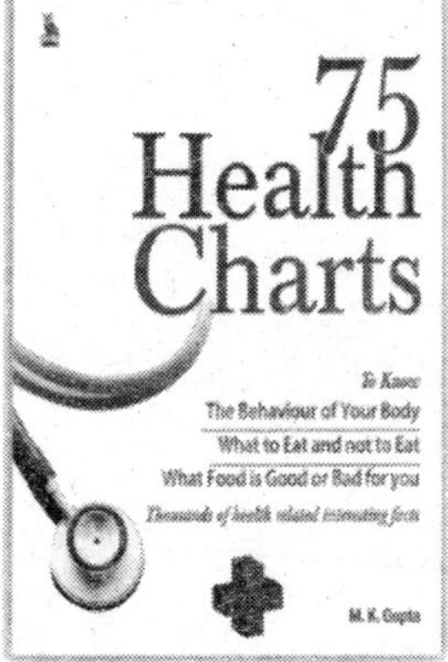

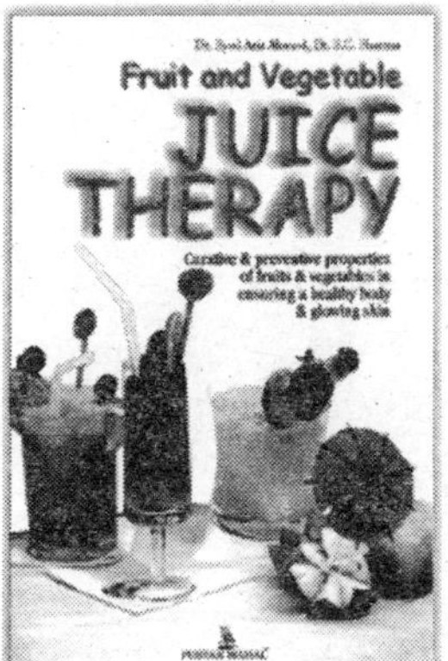

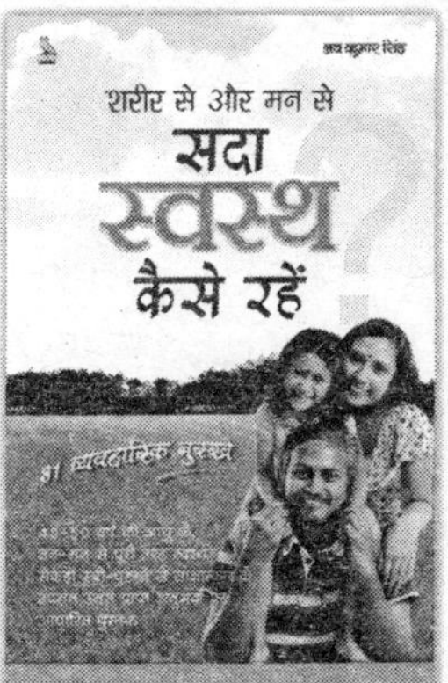

Postage Rs. 25/- each book.Every subsequent book: Rs. 5/- extra